Beyond Soap, Water, and Comb

A MAN'S GUIDE TO GOOD GROOMING AND FITNESS

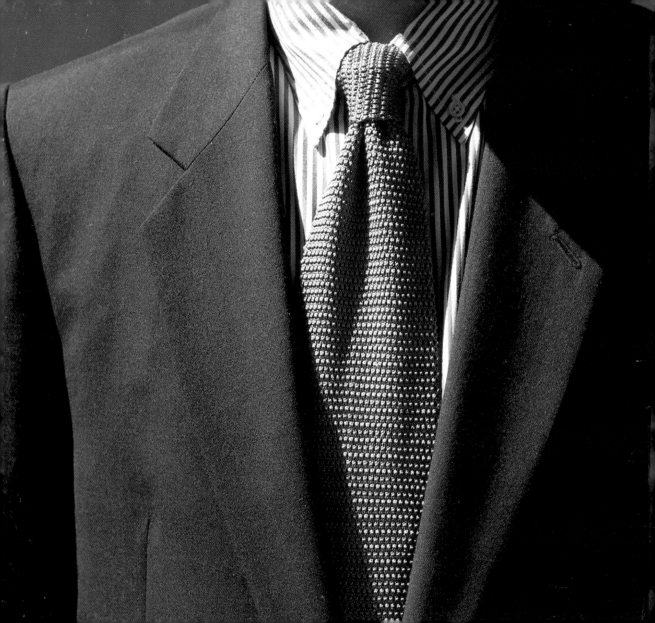

Beyond Soap, Water, and Comb

A MAN'S GUIDE TO GOOD GROOMING AND FITNESS

By Ed Marquand

Photography by Marsha Burns

ABBEVILLE PRESS PUBLISHERS
New York   London   Paris

DEDICATION This book is dedicated to my father. A fine role model of basic good grooming and a sensible, conservative wardrobe, he is amused that I have written this book. To both of us, memories of the haircut fights, wardrobe wars, and grooming disputes we had when I was a teenager are still too vivid, though several decades distant. But it was lessons before and since those difficult days that had as much influence on me as the barbershop battles.

Thanks, Dad.

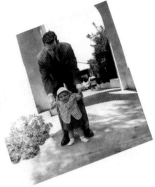

Text copyright © 1998 Ed Marquand. Photographs copyright © 1998 Marsha Burns except pages 5, 20, 24, 28, 30 bottom, 32, 39, 43, 45, 49, 97, 102 bottom, 107 left, 108 bottom, 112 bottom, 114, 117, 121 right, 122 top left & bottom right, 126, 131, 135, 137, 139, and 143 left, copyright © 1998 Ed Marquand. Compilation, including selection of text and images, copyright © 1998 Abbeville Press and Ed Marquand. All rights reserved under international copyright conventions. No part of this book may be reproduced or utilized in any form or by any means, including photocopying, recording, or by any information storage and retrieval system, without permission in writing from the publisher. Inquiries should be addressed to Abbeville Publishing Group, 22 Cortlandt Street, New York, NY 10007. The text of this book was set in Electra, Letter Gothic, and DIN Mittleschrift. Printed in Singapore.

First edition
10 9 8 7 6 5 4 3 2 1

Editor: Meredith Wolf Schizer; Designer: Gretchen Scoble; Production Director: Hope Koturo

Library of Congress Cataloging-in-Publication Data
Marquand, Ed.
     Beyond soap, water, and comb ; a man's guide to good grooming and fitness / by Ed Marquand ;
     photographs by Marsha Burns.
          p. cm.
     Includes index.
     ISBN 0-7892-0445-2
     1. Grooming for men. 2. Physical fitness for men. 3. Beauty, Personal. 4. Body image. I. Title.
RA777.8.M365 1998
646.7'044-dc21   98-12419

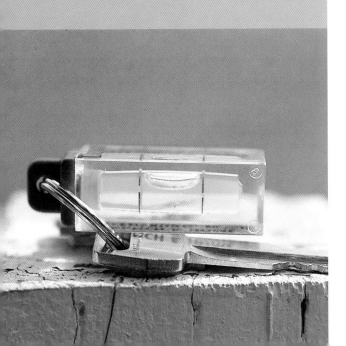

Table of
Contents

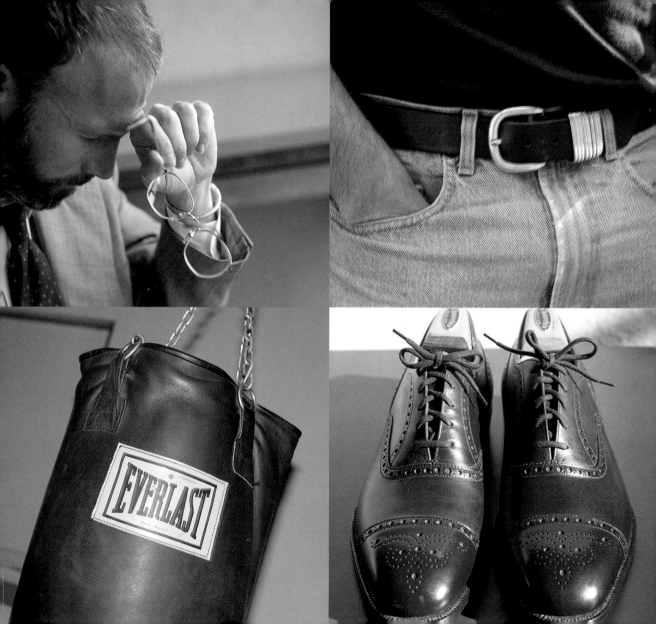

Preface

Stress clings to most men like mud to waffle boots—and it's just as hard to shed. Accumulated stress can affect your appearance, how you feel physically, and how you behave emotionally. Grooming, dressing, and taking good care of yourself should not cause anxiety; basic rituals of daily life should be fast, pleasurable, and easy. This book encourages you to understand and use classic, tried and true techniques to enhance your looks, confidence, and health.

The first part of this book takes your body—head to toe, scalp to sole—and reviews the best, most basic ways to groom it. Good grooming, confidence, and a natural appearance are a healthy combination, one that can be even more attractive than natural physical beauty.

If you can look good in jeans and a T-shirt, you can look great in all your clothes. An important feature of chapter 1 uses these two simple clothing items to help you set your fitness goals. Chapter 2 suggests simple ways to revise your diet and exercise plans to meet those goals.

The third chapter offers simple ways to improve your wardrobe and to develop a practical perspective on shopping, dressing, and caring for your clothes. Men can dress well without spending a fortune. Evaluate the clothes you have and those you need. Build and take care of a good, basic wardrobe, and enjoy the confidence of a man who dresses well.

Stress can be brutal to a guy. Chapter 4 offers ways to recharge emotionally. By examining the role, symptoms, and effects of stress, you can take better control of your life.

An appendix provides essential information about staying healthy. Basic medical advice—including critical warning signals—will help you keep track of your own vital signs.

By taking the simple advice and suggestions in this book, you should be able to live a happier, healthier, and more successful life.

Checkup and Maintenance

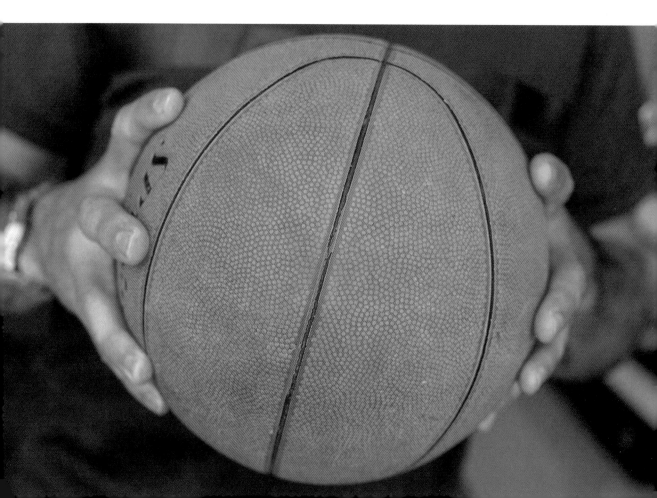

Getting a Grip

A quick look at the passing scene—or perhaps in the mirror—proves the need for this book. As I travel throughout the United States and abroad, I notice men—many of them successful business-men, others modern-day Willy Lomans—marching to their next meeting, to their next trade show, or on their way back home. Some of them look great. They carry themselves with an easy confidence. They appear fresh, alert, and engaged. A few have a distinct style or a taste for expensive fashion; many others look just fine in simple, basic clothes available in shops and malls anywhere.

But many of the guys I pass in airport terminals, on the sidewalks, or in shuttles to distant rental car lots need help. They look uncomfortable, insecure, awkward, tired, and older than they are. Many seem blind to their appearance, with no sense of a public self. Some look as if they slept in their clothes, or are wearing someone else's. Others look as if they have just maxed out their credit cards at a bad Miami haberdashery. But mostly they look as if they groomed and dressed in the dark and didn't glance at a mirror before leaving the house.

This phenomenon is more noticeable in the United States, sad to say. In general, European men (and there are many exceptions) are a little more self-aware and seem to get more of a kick out of the way they look. They aren't prissy—far from it. They just seem to have a better sense of themselves, and to take more pride in their appearance. As a rule, older Italian, French, or Spanish men look great, "normal," and classically confident. It doesn't take them hours to primp and fuss in front of their mirrors, nor have they spent fortunes on fashion. Still, they carry themselves with poise, grace, and confidence. They act as though they look much younger, and as though they add to the passing scene.

This is not to say that Americans are not capable of impressive fashion sense. Examples of glorious male display can be found all across America, in boardrooms, at truck stops, on Venice Beach, and in strip malls in Alabama. But as a whole, an attractive manliness is the exception, not the rule, though it can be achieved without a major wardrobe overhaul—or a personality transplant.

According to an overwhelming number of marketing surveys, psychological tests, and advertising focus groups, women perceive personal style in different ways than do men. There are fundamental differences between the way men and women see themselves. Women, according to this research, groom for each other and are extremely sensitive to the effect they create. Distinction is key; individuality is everything.

Men, on the other hand, find comfort in conformity. We opt for simplicity and basic acceptance by other men in our stylistic choices. Even though it is much easier for a guy to build a great wardrobe and spiff himself up than it is for a woman, too many men neglect even these basics in favor of a lazy carelessness that makes them look clueless more than comfortable.

You can look and feel great. You can simplify your life. You can be more attractive and successful. Just adopt the positive, healthy, and simple approach of this book.

Vanity vs. Self-confidence

Most men want to look good but don't want to worry about or work at it. Women, on the other hand, are willing to devote considerable time and energy to their appearance. For men, looking good doesn't always come easy—although it should and can. The key is confidence, grooming, health, and a few easy-to-follow tips.

Mirror-staring is unattractive on anyone, man or woman, no matter how goodlooking. The dance between self-confidence and unbearable vanity is a tricky one, but it can be learned. Here are some of the steps:

- Basic good grooming and fitness is about health, not vanity.

- To feel better, learn to take better care of yourself; when you feel better, you look better.

- Make your life habits a little healthier and more positive, and your body a little stronger. The payoff will be apparent to you and your friends.

- Time—today's most valuable commodity—is short. Design your grooming and fitness routines to be fast, efficient, and effective so they are easy to maintain.

- Dressing well should be simple.

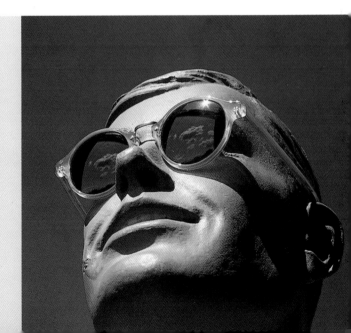

T-shirt Fit

The covers of men's magazines make it clear what most men want—a six-pack of abs. But for most of us that's like wanting to be three inches (7.6 cm) taller—it ain't gonna happen. Why are abs so important? Perhaps they represent ultimate fitness: if you have great abs, the rest of you is likely to be buffed too. But unless you do sit-ups for a living, abs that good are a fantasy. Instead, let's set a goal of looking good in jeans and a T-shirt. That's possible. Not easy, perhaps, but at least plausible.

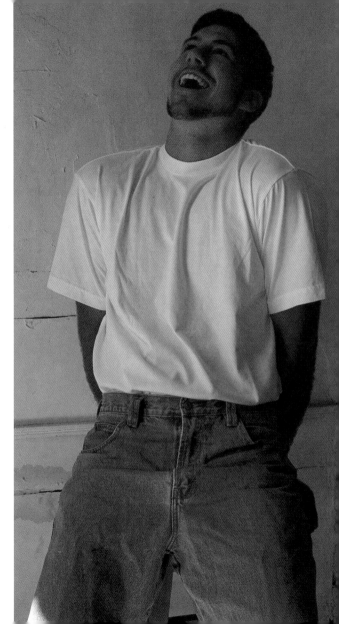

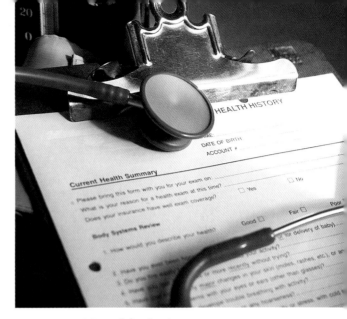

FIRST, MAKE AN APPOINTMENT FOR A PHYSICAL. Most of this book presumes your fundamental good health. Since you are ultimately responsible for your health, get a physical exam every few years. The younger you are, the less frequently you need one, but don't neglect your health, and learn to monitor your basic functions. The appendix (pages 150–57) provides basic medical advice and the major early warning signs of potential problems. Make use of this information.

If it's been more than two years since your last physical, call your doctor and schedule one. Getting a clean bill of health is a great way to eliminate a big chunk of lurking anxiety. If it takes several weeks to get an appointment, use this time to improve your habits and fitness routines before the doctor sees you.

THEN, GET THE BIG PICTURE. Have you ever been surprised by the way you look in a snap-shot or a video? It is hard to be objective about the way others see you if you only know yourself as a bleary face in the shaving mirror each morning. To look and feel your best you need an accurate self-image—a big, three-dimensional picture of your public self.

Sure, this can be discouraging at first, but don't despair. You need a starting point. Any fitness coach will tell you that the further you have to go, the more quickly you will notice a big improvement.

How do you get a clear big picture? Take pictures. Polaroids, snapshots taken by a friend or partner (or a self-timer), even a video. You may feel extremely self-conscious, but it will be worth every pang of embarrassment. You can also start with a full-length and a hand mirror to examine your body and to look at your sides or back.

Check yourself out wearing casual clothes you most often wear. Overall, how do you look? Okay? Or like some slob you'd see hunkered down in a bus station? How do the clothes fit? Are they too tight or too loose? Do you look sharp or dressed for moving day? Stylish or random? Even more than your physique, your clothes give you away. Simple changes can make a big difference (see Wardrobe Basics, pages 71–91).

Few men are ever satisfied with their physiques: it's hard to look great in a Speedo. But there's a big difference between looking good on the street and knocking them out on the beach. Since the goal is to look better in jeans and a T-shirt, that's what you should put on now.

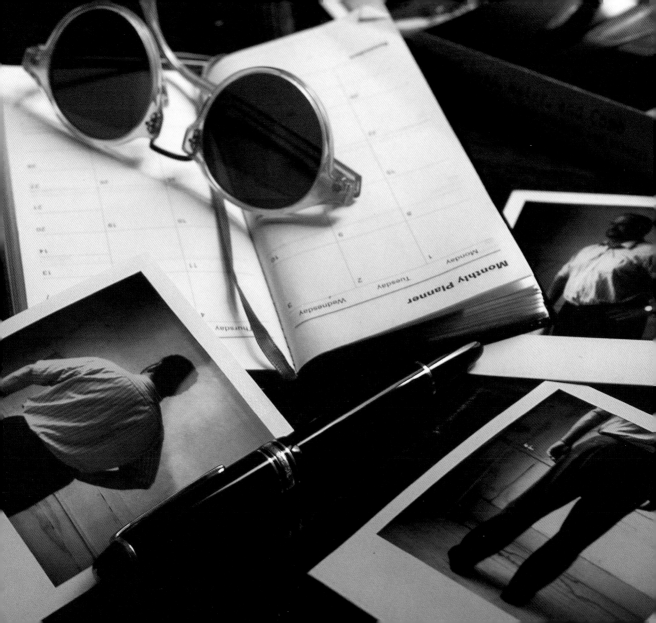

JEANS AND A T-SHIRT: It's a classic American look. Maybe you'll never look like Brando at his peak, but you can look better than you do today. And if you can look good in jeans and a T-shirt, you can look great in most other clothes. Instead of fixating on measurements and weight, we are going to use these two pieces of clothing as your standard. You can use them to measure your progress. Take these easy steps:

- Put on a pair of jeans and a T-shirt (tucked in) that you want to wear, but that are a little too tight—or too loose, if you are trying to gain weight. They shouldn't be new, because you don't want them to shrink. (Even broken-in cotton keeps shrinking with repeated washings.) Put on the kind of underpants you typically wear. No need for a belt.

- Face the mirror and look at yourself honestly. Stand up straight. Now relax. Is the waist too tight? By how much? If the jeans are way too tight, your goals might be too ambitious. Get another pair of jeans.

- Do you have the wrong kind of six-pack on your abs? Shoulders slouching? Major love handles? No evident muscle tone? Take it all in. You are establishing the starting point right here and now.

- Imagine what would change if you were 5-10 percent more fit than you are today. What would it look like? What would you change? Fix on that image. Write a quick description of what you see and feel, and what you would eventually like to see and feel. In listing your goals, be specific with each part.

- Date your notes. Write down weights and measurements if you like. Fold the note up and put it in your pocket. When you are finished, take off your T-shirt and jeans. Fold them and put them someplace out of the way. Sure, you won't be able to wear them for a while, but that's a small sacrifice for the help it will provide.

- In a month, try on these two items again. These clothes will not lie to you, and they reveal and reinforce your efforts simply and effectively.

- Make this a monthly ritual, on the same day (or weekend) each month. Continue after you reach your goals to remind you of the habits that helped get you there.

- If your goal is to lose lots of weight, and you succeed to where your pants are as baggy a clown's, keep switching to a smaller size that feels snug to help you keep on target.

HOW DO YOU LOOK? HOW DO YOU FEEL? The jeans-and-a-T-shirt exercise has helped you get the big picture. Now let's review how you look and feel every day. Identify all of your problem areas and establish a routine for improvement. Create a checklist and review your progress every month or so. Like a workout sheet in a gym, this makes it easier to see steady progress. If you are so inclined, you can add physical measurements, but don't get carried away with details. Remember, focus on the broad strokes; you are trying to get a good overview first, and details can come later.

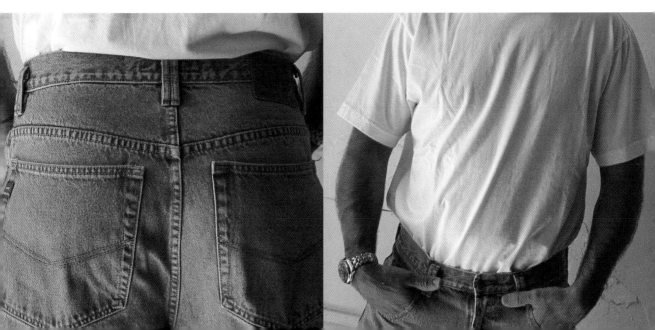

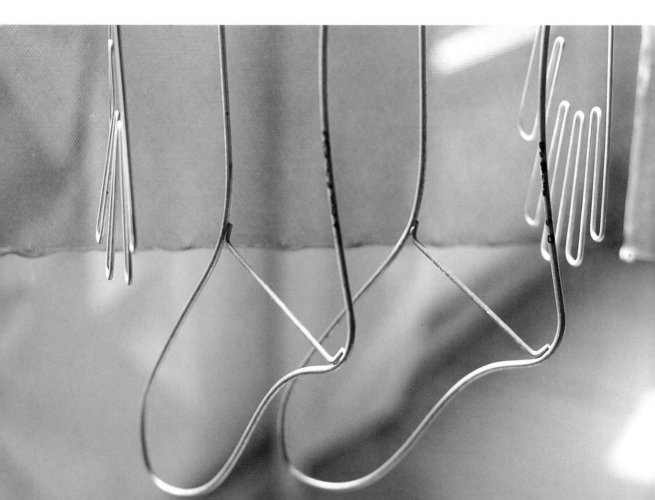

Your Head

Men spend too much time staring forlornly in the mirror and worrying about losing their hair. Instead, they should take good care of what they've got and move south to the rest of their bodies. Although follicles age at a genetically determined rate, you can make sure you don't speed that rate by abusing your hair or scalp. Here are some pointers so that every day can be a good hair day:

- Treat your hair and your scalp properly.

- Make sure you eat properly and get enough water.

- Avoid sun- and windburn.

- Some bleaches and dyes can harm vulnerable, sputtering hair follicles, so think twice before deciding to become a bottle blond.

- Be wary of products that gradually darken gray hair; they may contain chemicals that are ultimately bad for you.

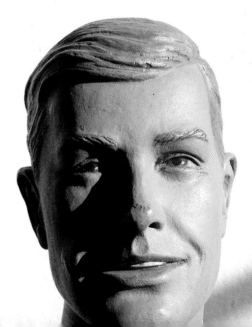

SHAMPOO BASICS: Clean hair signals general good hygiene, but don't over-shampoo. If your hair is dry, every other day with just a daily rinse should be fine.

- If you have ever tried to shampoo with bar soap, you've probably ended up with gunkier hair than when you started. Shampoo cuts through oils and grease more effectively than bar soap.

- Spend a few minutes reading and comparing shampoo labels, and buy a basic product balanced for the quality and texture of your hair. It doesn't need to be expensive.

- Wet your hair thoroughly so that your hair is soaked completely before applying shampoo.

- Use just enough shampoo to clean well. Don't overscrub. Work up lather with a slow, firm, gentle massage for a long minute. Work your scalp muscles and let yourself enjoy this brief ritual.

- Unless you work on an oil rig (or your hair is extraordinarily oily), you probably don't need to wash twice, whatever the bottle instructions say.

- Use a conditioner once or twice a week to keep your hair from getting overly dried out. Overconditioned hair looks flat.

- Beef up thinning hair slightly with thickening shampoos. They do add bulk to each strand, so it will make your hair look thicker.

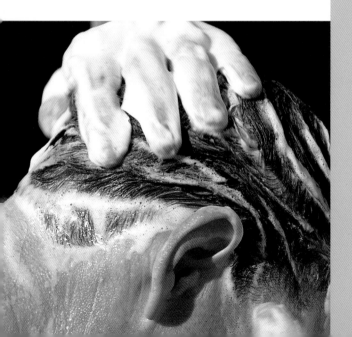

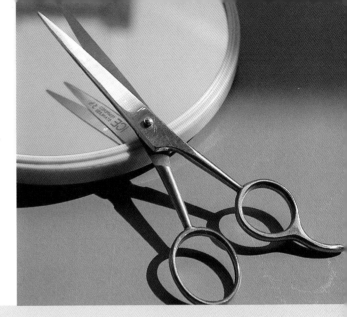

SNOW JOB: A little dandruff and flaky skin is normal, but heavy snowfall can be caused by many things: bad scalp care, poor circulation, inadequate rinsing, the wrong shampoo, excessive scratching, stress, skin problems, sunburn, poor diet, dehydration, dry air, vitamin deficiency, or a more serious condition or infection.

- Most flaky skin is not caused by infectious dandruff, so dandruff shampoos may not be the best remedy. If you suffer from this problem, start with the simple solutions first —like more careful shampooing and rinsing—before subjecting yourself to more aggressive treatments.

- Stop scratching your head. That alone may take care of the problem. Shampoo more carefully and gently massage your soapy scalp for a full minute to increase circulation. Rinse your hair more thoroughly. If that doesn't do it, eliminate hair tonics, gels, or mousses. Within a week or two, you should notice an improvement.

- If you are still flaking, switching shampoos is the next step; pH-neutral brands may be better suited to your skin chemistry. Try that for another week or two.

- If these solutions fail, you may have more serious skin trouble that requires a dandruff shampoo or professional medical attention.

GET A GOOD HAIRCUT: A good haircut indicates high self-esteem. Some men really do look great in a basic crew cut, but most men look spiffier with a little more professional tonsorial attention. Find a barber or stylist who knows what she is doing—someone you enjoy going to. A trip to the barber should be more fun than going to the dentist.

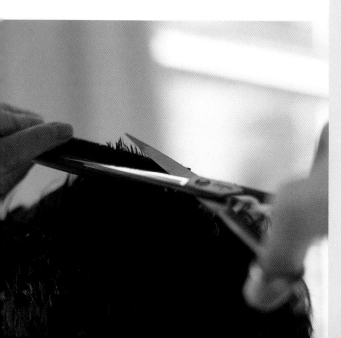

- A bad haircut never looks good. A good haircut looks great when it is freshly cut, as it grows in, and as it grows long. You shouldn't need to make weekly trips for trims—in fact, you may be able to get away with four or even six weeks between visits—but don't make a trip to the hairstylist an annual event.

- If you doubt the ability or taste of the person who currently cuts your hair, ask someone who always has a good haircut for a recommendation.

- What looks terrific on George Clooney or Harrison Ford might not be right for you. A good hairstylist gets to know you, your head, and the cut that will complement your head shape, facial structure, and overall look.

- When you get your hair cut, bring pictures of friends or cut from magazines showing haircuts that you like. Ask your barber or stylist if a similar style might flatter you as well.

- If you shower twice in the day, and you don't have time to fuss with blow-dryers, ask for a haircut that looks fine wet or dry.

HAIR CREDIBILITY: Dye jobs, rugs, and plugs—who are you kidding? Even the models in the ads don't look convincing. Maybe those products work for some movie actors, but the actors have stylists primping between takes. If you saw them in person, their hair might seem less flattering.

This is one area where vanity signals get loud and out of control. Unfortunately, hair credibility depends on the successful balance of skin tone, color, eyebrow color, thickness and texture of surrounding hair, age, haircut, and lots of high maintenance. Difficult to keep in balance, each of these factors can be a tip-off that you're faking it.

HAIR COLORING: The hair tones men often end up with, especially when they rely on over-the-counter stuff, can get spooky. And given all the strange lighting conditions where we live, a dye job that looks great in a hair salon can turn purple or orange under natural light outside, or under fluorescent lights at the gym. Once it looks fake to your friends, that's how they will remember it.

Women wear colored hair better than men, and are willing to pay more for professional help. And if you are thinking of adjusting your hair color, have it done professionally—*every few weeks!* On average, your hair grows half an inch (1.25 cm) per month—and roots are tough to hide.

RUGS: Toupees occasionally help some men's appearance, but not usually. If you do wear one, and have no intention of losing it, buy an expensive one, wear it well, have it professionally tended, and get adjoining hair cut regularly.

PLUGS: Plugs—hair follicles transferred from some other part of your body—are just too bizarre for most men to consider. Perhaps some day scientists will find a way to make them look less agricultural. They have a long way to go.

Going bald can be just fine, if you surrender to the inevitable. Cut what you have nicely, and focus on the other 99.9 percent of your body.

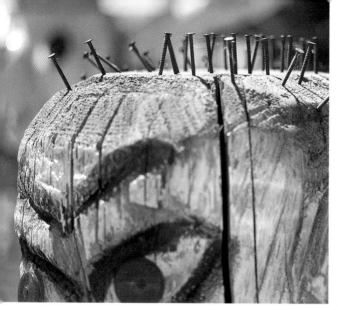

BALDING BASICS: Genetically, you are programmed to keep your hair for only so many years before your follicles start to sputter and shut down. If you are lucky and come from rare stock that keeps nice thick heads of hair into old age, count your blessings. But if genetics is working against that, or if stress, poor nutrition, chemical exposure, or hormonal changes cause you to lose your hair earlier than you'd like, trying to prevent baldness is like trying to stop leaves from falling from a tree in autumn.

Some guys go bald as early as high school and still look terrific. Keep in mind: your hair is a bigger deal to you than it is to anyone else, and all you have to do is look around at the many examples of good-looking guys who are balding to see how little it needs to affect a man's entire image. You can save yourself lots of time, trouble, and psychic energy by making the best of what you have while you have it and accepting its loss gracefully.

NEW DRUGS: Pharmaceutical companies are hell-bent on creating the perfect drug to prevent balding. But these drugs have drawbacks, which you should consider before succumbing to their consequences. First, they are expensive. Second, they don't always work. Third, they can affect other parts of your body—including your libido—in unexpected ways. Finally, you may have to take them for the rest of your days; once you stop taking them, your hair may retreat.

HOLDING ON TO WHAT YOU HAVE: Don't smoke cigars or cigarettes. Eat right. Don't drink too much alcohol, but drink plenty of water. Get enough sleep. Treat your scalp and hair properly. Avoid bleaches, dyes, and weird chemicals. Don't get sunburned (wear sunblock on your scalp and any exposed skin). Avoid temperature and humidity extremes for long stretches. Get a good haircut, and wear what you have proudly. Resort to pharmaceuticals only if you are desperate, but be aware of the possible downsides: a lifelong prescription and a possible decline of sex drive.

GETTING RID OF HAIR WHERE YOU DON'T WANT IT: It's sad irony for many men that the only place on their bodies they can't grow enough hair is their scalps, but life can be tough that way. If you want to remove body hair temporarily, you can clip, shave, wax, pluck, or chemically strip off hair. More permanent laser and electrolysis techniques are also available, though at a much higher price. Any of the following techniques should work for most body hair, but experiment first with the technique that you plan to use to make sure you aren't going to be disappointed or uncomfortable with the results.

CLIPPING: For most men who are not swimmers, bodybuilders, or porn stars, hair is a fact of life. If you look more like a beast than a man, perhaps you can cut back much of your body hair so that more of your skin can show through. With a pair of scissors, standing in front of the mirror, start on your chest and take a few light (very light) swipes. Does it look better? Keep going then. If not, stop there and reconsider.

TIP: *Don't clog up the drain on your washbasin. First, plug the drain and keep the sink dry. When you are through, wipe out the sink with your hand and throw the trimmings in the trash. Get the rest of the hair with a damp paper towel or tissue.*

SHAVING: Shaving only lops off fur at skin level, so like a lawn, it will grow back all too soon. Still, this may be the best, cheapest, fastest, and simplest method for most men. But one result you should know about before heading into virgin forest is that if you shave too close, the hair may regrow down rather than out, and you could suffer ingrown hairs. Also, any area of your skin covered by clothes will feel different and may itch, almost like rough wool.

If smooth perfection is too much trouble— you don't mind hair, but you don't want *so much*—some men find that a quick, light pass with a dry razor, barely grazing the skin, is a good way to hack back fur patches on the back, shoulders, or chest so they are less obvious. This reduces chances for ingrown hair, and is quick, clean, inexpensive, and effective. Your clothes may feel strange on your skin until you adjust to the new sensation, though.

WAXING AND SUGARING: Women have been waxing and peeling their body hair for decades now, and you can too—for back or chest hair in particular, although the technique will work anywhere. (Let vanity and your threshold for pain be your guide.) Essentially, your skin is lathered with warmed wax or a sheet of sticky sugar. The emulsion attaches itself to your hairs, and with a quick yank, they are pulled out by the root. It can be painful—you've pulled bandages off before, you know the sensation. Some areas are more sensitive than others, so it's your call. Hair does grow back in six to eight weeks, and if your hair is tight and curly, you may have trouble with ingrown hairs. You can do this with over-the-counter products or have it done professionally. Your hairstylist or barber may be able to recommend a good practitioner.

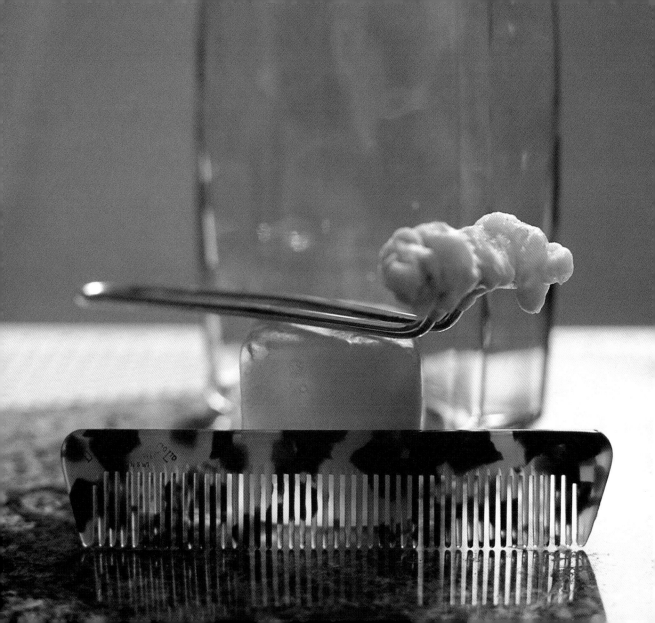

PLUCKING: The patient man's—or masochist's—peel. With a good pair of tweezers, you can go at the task one hair at a time, but the hair will grow back, and you can damage your hair follicle. Still, for eyebrows, ears, and around moles, this method may be for you.

TIP: *Numb the area to be plucked by running an ice cube over the skin for a minute or so first.*

ELECTROLYSIS: This method is best for small areas of particularly annoying and visible hair. Women often use it to remove potential mustaches and for eyebrow styling. With electrolysis, hair will grow back, but after a few treatments—and it may take a several—most of the follicles give up. This technique can be expensive, and it can permanently damage the skin in the treated areas. If you go this route, check out professional references.

LASER REMOVAL: This technique can permanently destroy follicles through heat exchange. It is pricey, and it will take several sessions to complete the task. Some sensitive skin may blister, and men with darker complexions may have less success with this method, as their hair tends to be tougher. Leave this to professionals also.

BACK HAIR: All these methods work, but the do-it-yourself methods require reach. It's foolish and dangerous to shave, pluck, or peel your own back, so you must rely on the kindness of partners, friends, or professionals.

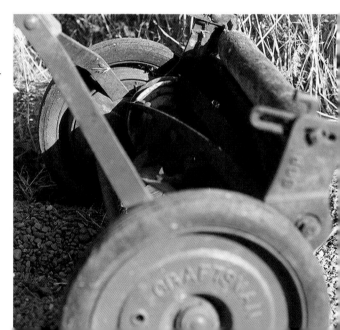

FACIAL HAIR POINTERS: Your eyebrows, eyelashes, beard, and mustache only require basic care too. Remember to shampoo them, and rinse well to avoid flaking. Follow your hairstylist's advice about the cut and style of your facial hair to make it suit your face and haircut. Trim your beard or mustache between visits to the barber. Use high-grade scissors, a fine comb, your razor, or clippers designed for the task. Your hairstylist can give you pointers.

SHAVING AND SAVING FACE: Shaving is more than an annoying morning ritual; it has an important effect on your skin tone and complexion. So do it properly.

- Shave after showering.

- Use quality shaving cream to help each whisker soak up water. Your options are many; pick a shaving cream that suits your skin type.

- Leave shaving cream on your face for at least one minute before shaving.

- Always use a sharp blade. Some men can get a week or two of good service out of a blade, but those with tougher beards go through them more quickly. When yours starts to pull, replace it.

- To prevent ingrown hairs, shave in the direction your beard grows.

- After each swipe, rinse the blade and remoisten the section you just shaved, spreading a thin layer of lather from another area of your face. Feel for areas that are still rough and shave them again. Keep everything moist.

- Don't overshave. You are only trying to cut your whiskers down to size, not rearrange your hair follicles. For good skin health, shave only as much as your razor easily allows.

- Rinse thoroughly. Use a dab of lotion to hold moisture in. Alcohol-based aftershaves do more harm than good.

- Easy on the cologne. If you use any at all—and many people find other people's cologne repulsive—keep it subtle. Very subtle. If you can still smell it strongly fifteen minutes after applying to your wrist or on your neck below your ears, you've used too much. And if you are heading for the gym, wash it off before your workout.

Basic skin care

Throughout your life your skin grows, ages, and replaces itself. A proper diet, drinking adequate water (six to eight glasses a day), avoiding drugs or excessive use of alcohol, protecting your skin from sunburn and exposure, and getting adequate sleep will ward off the ravages of aging far better than any expensive goop.

Major department stores have discovered big money in male cosmetics. The advertising

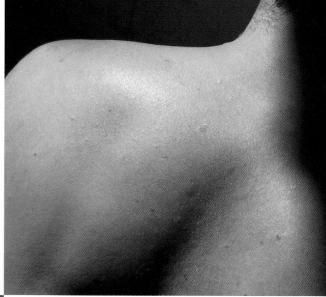

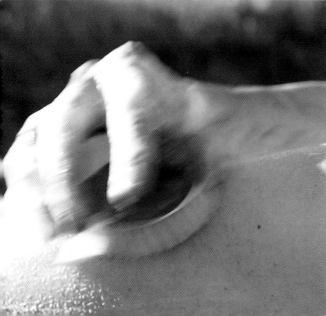

pressure is fierce. Not only are most of the products absurdly expensive and complicated to use, but most of them make unsupportable claims to rejuvenate, restore, and repair damaged flesh. This is advertising over science and reason. Unless you really enjoy the indulgence of facial rituals or have serious skin trouble, find a good soap to clean your skin and the right moisturizer to retain more natural moisture, and be done with all of the cosmetic nonsense.

PROTECTING YOUR FACE AGAINST
WIND, RAIN, AND FIRE. Protect first.
Prevent skin from damage with sunblock and
moisturizers. Once the damage is done, all
you can do is disguise your damaged skin. By
applying cream, you are filling tiny cracks,
almost like waxing a car, so your skin only
looks better.

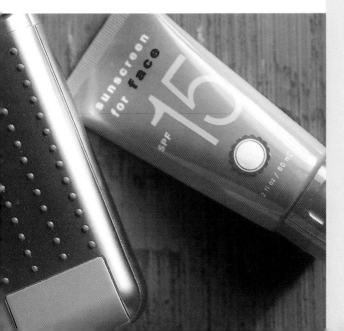

- Sun and wind are brutal; take skin cancer
  warnings seriously. Only a few decades ago,
  common wisdom said it was okay to burn and
  peel at the beginning of every summer, so long
  as you eventually tanned. True—to a point. Some
  studies have shown that vacationing professionals
  who suffer severe sunburn do more harm to their
  skin in a few days than farmers who spend most
  of the year in the sunshine. But the burn/heal
  approach is foolish, as generations of skin cancer
  victims now realize. The steady depletion of the
  ozone has made it even more important now to
  protect against ultraviolet (UV) rays .

- Not all sunscreens are up to the task, and no
  sunscreen will completely eliminate the risk of
  the skin cancer melanoma, basal cell carcinoma,
  and squamous cell carcinoma. Use one that
  blocks both UVA and UVB rays, with at least
  15 SPF (sun protection factor) for daily exposure,
  and 20 to 30 SPF for strong sunlight. Put sunscreen
  on at least fifteen minutes before exposure. The
  best protection is to cover your skin, wear a hat,
  and avoid exposure in the middle of the day. Pale
  vacationers and fair-skinned, blue-eyed people
  with a family history of melanoma should take
  special precaution.

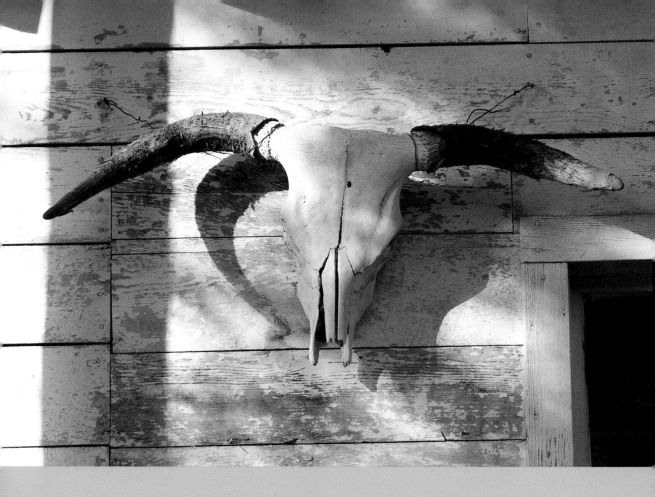

SKIN SKINNY—DEALING WITH SKIN PROBLEMS: Other than infections or systemic medical problems, most skin problems are matters of moisture—your skin is too oily or it is too dry. Raging hormones in adolescence trigger excess oil production. These oils accumulate and get infected in budding oil glands to produce typical teenage acne. It can be brutal for some guys. Some over-the-counter acne treatments can help, but serious cases should be checked out by a dermatologist. Wash frequently with a mild soap. Do not scrub. Benzoyl peroxide gel or cream can be effective if used properly. Read and follow the instructions for these products carefully.

By your mid-twenties these hormonal surges have settled down, and some stability is achieved. Healthy skin can be maintained simply by regular washing with soap and water. For normal skin, you don't need to scrub, peel, or exfoliate. Regular washing with the right soap and gentle cleaning with a washcloth is plenty.

Not all soaps are good for your face, particularly if you have sensitive skin. Obviously, lava soaps designed to clean heavy grease off your hands are not good for your face—or the rest of your body. But even some basic brand soaps are chemically rougher than you'd think. pH-neutral soaps are gentler, clean without drying out your skin unnecessarily, and may solve typical skin problems. Rinse thoroughly. Soapy residue can continue to dry your skin for hours after washing, absorbing essential oils and creating a layer that interferes with your natural daily skin processes.

STEROID STUPIDITY: If you are tempted to take steroids, figure on big-time acne and other skin problems brought on by exaggerated hormonal output. You may think others will find your new buffness attractive, but the side effects won't be. Steroids should never be used without professional medical supervision. Other side effects can include baldness, decreased sex drive, shrunken testicles, and dangerous mood swings.

PATCHY SKIN: If your diet is good but your skin is still patchy, flaky, or too dry, try switching soaps before self-treating yourself with medicinal creams. Start with a pH-balanced brand for a few weeks. Even expensive, "hypoallergenic" brands may not work for you, so experiment until you find one that suits your skin. If that doesn't take care of the problem, move on to more aggressive medicinal treatments.

COSMETIC SURGERY: For the desperate or the deeply insecure, cosmetic surgery offers hope, but nothing about surgery is simple or without consequences. Skin that has been surgically altered doesn't always age at the same rate as the skin around it. Gravity pulls and changes the way flesh drapes, so after a few years your reupholstery begins to look odd and unnatural. Even a quick look through a celebrity magazine will reveal the up- and the downsides of plastic surgery. Some male movie stars look like bad wax mannequins of themselves. Others have that deer-in-the-headlights look. As with hair color, women have an easier time disguising the imperfections with makeup. Men don't usually want to commit themselves to that kind of camouflage.

THE ALLURE OF LIPOSUCTION: Who wouldn't want to vacuum away extra fat? The problem is that it is difficult to isolate fat from blood vessels and nerves, so it's easy for parts you want to keep to get sucked up in the soup. To be fair, many men have enjoyed the benefits of plastic surgery and liposuction, and techniques improve every year, but if there are other ways to achieve the body of your dreams— or if you can grow to like the face you were meant to have—you may be sparing yourself unfortunate and unintended consequences.

Calibrating your instruments: eyes, ears, and nose

EYES: Beyond protecting them, they don't need much care.

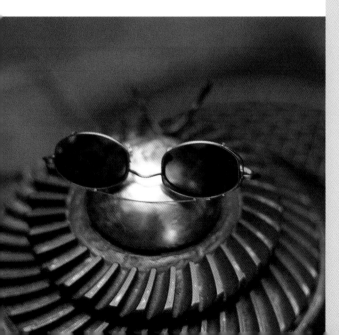

- Unless you have a specific problem, you need to visit an ophthalmologist only every two years for a full checkup. If you notice a decline in your vision, don't fret, but get it checked. As we age, our lenses harden and aren't as pliable, so they take longer to focus. Men may take this as unnatural or unusual, but it's a nearly universal phenomenon. Eye exercises may help for some problems, but not for general aging or hardening of the lenses.

- If you wear glasses, keep your prescription current.

- Buy some spiffy glass frames that work with your face and personal style. There are some terrific designs, some of them are incredibly lightweight and comfortable. These days, many men really do look better in glasses.

- Some vision problems can be permanently corrected with laser eye surgery. Although the techniques are relatively new, many men are finding the results much more satisfying than glasses or contact lenses. Any surgery involves risk, so research your options thoroughly.

- Contact lenses need careful cleaning, so follow your doctor's instructions. To prevent eye infections, do not moisten lenses with saliva. Your mouth is crawling with germs you don't want swimming around in your eyes.

- Don't rub your eyes. Keep your fingers out of them.

- Wear UV-filtering sunglasses in bright sun and protective eyewear when you work with tools or in dusty or potentially toxic locations.

- Don't rely on steady doses of eye drops to keep your eyes clear and moist. If they are often dry, you may not be drinking enough water or getting enough sleep, or your tear ducts may not be functioning properly. Have an ophthalmologist check them out.

- Eye strain can be exhausting and counterproductive. Be sure to look up from your work—especially close-up work or at your computer—every fifteen minutes or so to give your eyes a chance to refocus and your eye muscles some rest. Let them unfocus for a few seconds, look out a window, or even across the room.

NOSE NEWS: Other than keeping drugs out of it, about the only maintenance a guy's nose needs is occasional nose hair trimming. Scissors with rounded tips, or little tubular grinders, are recommended. You are not trying for sinus reconstruction here, so don't trim any deeper than you can easily see in a mirror.

CAN YOU EAR ME? Good grooming aside, your ears are far more delicate and sensitive to loud noise than you may realize. A steady dose of power tools, car alarms, sirens, loudspeakers, lawnmowers, engines, hammering, and loud music—especially from headsets and concerts—can actually destroy the fibers inside your ear canals. And they don't grow back. Get a hearing test, and you may be surprised how many frequencies you can no longer hear. It's a

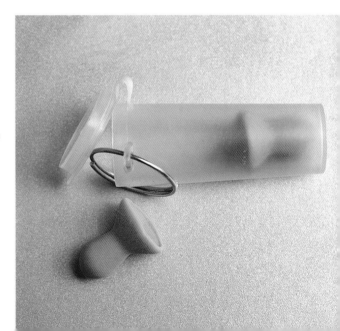

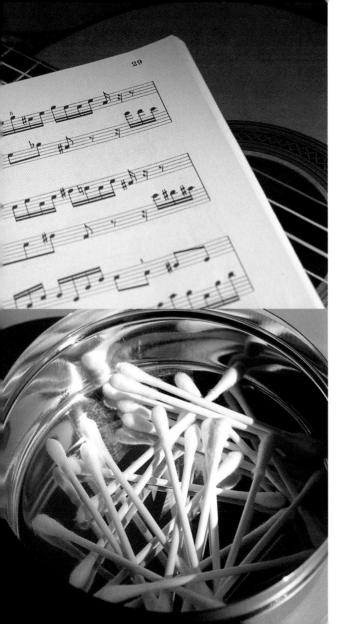

little depressing, but instructive, and it may help you realize how important it is to hold on to what you haven't yet wasted. Besides, asking "Huh?" all the time isn't attractive to anyone old enough to vote.

Scrub behind your ears, like Mom always said, but do it carefully. She also should have told you never to stick anything smaller than your index finger into your ear, and even then, make sure it's clean. Q-tips, warm water, and mild soap can keep the outer ear clean, but if you suspect that wax buildup is cutting down on your hearing, use an over-the-counter solution to help soften and remove it. If your ear hair is becoming bushy, trim it.

Watch your mouth:
keeping your teeth, gums, and tongue healthy

Healthy teeth are a gift of our time. With fluoridated water, tooth decay and fillings are no longer an automatic rite of passage. But you still need to brush to prevent decay, and your gums need a good massage from brushing or flossing at least twice a day to keep them firm and pink, with good circulation. Flossing catches the food that gets caught between your teeth and removes the ingredients that build up into plaque.

It is important to take care of your teeth throughout your life so they can continue to serve you into ripe old age. Tooth decay is most likely to affect younger men. By the time you are in your thirties, though, gum problems may appear, and great teeth in bad gums isn't a good combination. In fact, if your gums recede far enough, your roots will show, making them more susceptible to decay and sensitive to temperature. Face it, you need to take good care of your teeth, gums, and mouth throughout your life.

Suck ice if you must, but don't chew it. The cold, pressure, and impact can create cracks and fissures in your teeth that will haunt your future.

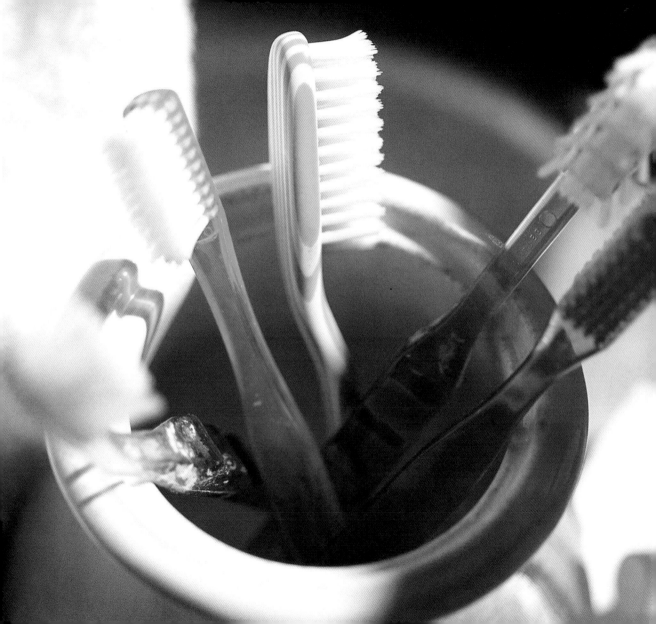

As for that spongy tongue of yours, you need to brush it too, because that's where lots of bad breath starts. If this is not part of your morning routine, try brushing your teeth as you normally would, and then rinse. Now brush your tongue with a little dab of toothpaste and spit. Chances are, you still had lots of gunk in your mouth that the first brushing didn't remove. That's the stuff that festers and creates bad breath. Get rid of it regularly, at least once a day. The farther back you can reach without gagging, the better. Pull from the back of the tongue to the front with the wide side of your toothbrush. With practice, it can feel good, and it will help keep good relations with the neighbors.

STOP SPITTING: Don't spit, period. It's rude, but it's also unsanitary. Many serious diseases throughout history, including tuberculosis, have been spread this way. Imagine tracking through someone else's saliva and spreading it around your living room carpet. Get the picture?

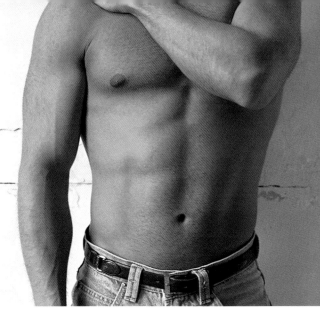

Your Torso

Now that we've covered your head, we can move south to the rest of your body.

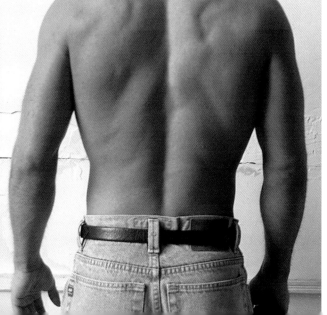

SKIN CARE, SUNBURN, AND MAINTAINING AND IMPROVING SKIN TONE: Though it has less of a public face, the skin on the rest of your body deserves to be treated well, too. Keep it clean, protect it from sunburn, and use a little moisturizer to help retain its natural moisture. Start with a good shower.

SHOWERS, HOT AND COLD: Few pleasures in life are as refreshing as a shower, so enjoy every moment. Buy a back brush. It feels great to dig into hard-to-reach spots and scrub, like a bear rubbing against the trunk of a tree. Sponges, washcloths, and loofahs make fine scrubbers too, but a good brush is unbeatable. Guys with back acne also benefit from good, regular scrubbing.

Some men swear by cold showers to get them going in the morning. Though they may feel good afterward, the shock they put your system through may not appeal to you. Try a blast some morning and see if the boost it gives your circulation is worth the chill.

Good as they feel, long showers can dry out sensitive skin by washing away your body's protective oils. While you shower, keep an eye out for rashes, warts, odd moles, or any evidence of skin cancer. It never hurts to do a quick check of your testicles too for unusual bumps or sensitivities.

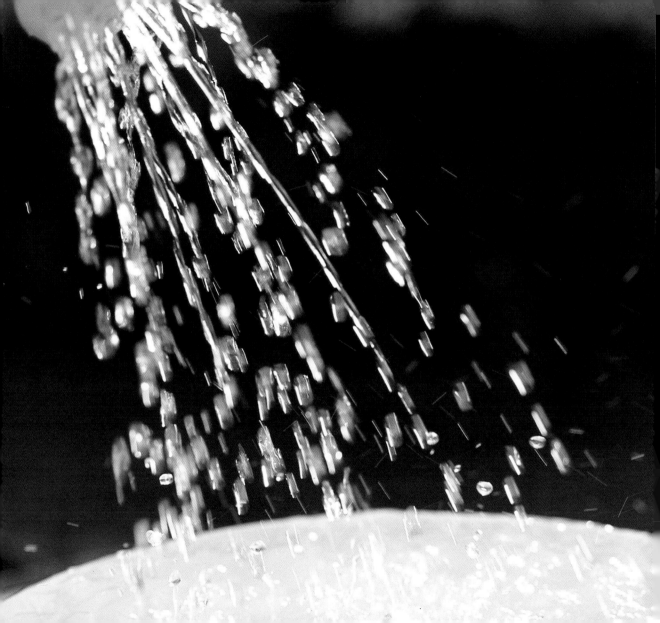

TANNING SALONS AND TANNING
LOTIONS: Raised under the influence of
Hollywood, we equate tanned skin with health
and beauty, and that is a hard notion to shake.
Pallid, cadaverous flesh can't compare with
images of toned, tropical bodies, bursting with
vigor and energy. But skin cancer is no picnic,
and unfortunately it is a real threat, particularly
to those with pale, sensitive skin and occasional
sunbathers—i.e. most of us.

Recently, dermatologists have questioned
the wisdom of exposing your skin to UV radia-
tion of any kind. The whole tanning salon
industry has been built on the notion that
certain UV rays are harmless, while others are
dangerous. Some experts now think that the
only safe UV ray is one that never reaches
your skin.

So what are the alternatives? There are
tanning lotions that chemically alter the pig-
ment of your skin. Sometimes they don't even
look orange, and they are probably safer than
tanning beds. Test them on small patches first.

REMOVING TATTOOS: Everyone makes
mistakes. Though possible to remove much
pigmentation by infrared coagulation, this is
not an easy process, and the results are uneven
depending on the location, skin tone, and
quality of the tattoo. Consult a dermatologist
regarding your specific regrets.

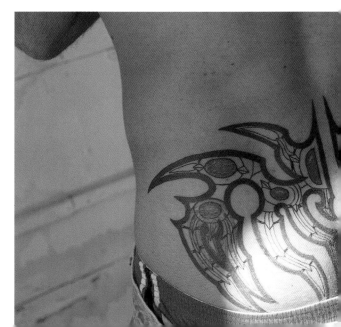

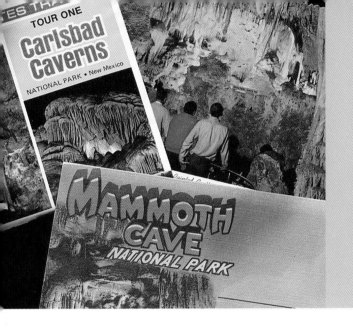

Where the sun doesn't shine: your pits, cracks, crevices, and crotch.

There are only a few places on your body where flesh meets flesh, and that's good—trouble can arise more quickly in those places. Hair, living and dead skin, glandular secretions, and bodily fluids team up to create mini-swamps, inadequately ventilated. You want them to be healthy wetlands, not toxic dumps. The basic rules about cleanliness apply here, but give them deliberate attention.

YOUR PITS: These intersections of arms and torso are important because of the variety of glands and lymph nodes lurking beneath the underarms. Feel around occasionally, as you should with your testicles, for signs of unusual or painful swelling. Unless you are under great stress and have been eating very heavily spiced foods, sweat, as such, doesn't smell so bad. But if it has a chance to mix with old sweat, dead skin, dirt, and residual bacteria, the odor can be choking.

As for cleaning, keep sweat glands clean and free flowing. Every shower, take your washcloth and soap—some common brands are antibacterial—and give your pits a good scrub. Let the soap lather up for at least ten seconds to ensure that the bacteria is good and dead. Rinse thoroughly. This may take care of most of the problem, and you may not need that super-duper deodorant after all. If you still smell riper than you should, dermatologists recommend taking small doses of zinc—25 to 50 milligrams—in tablet form every day.

Most antiperspirants contain chemicals that shut down your sweat glands, but this may not be a good idea over time. Common sense tells us that these pieces of microplumbing may be performing an important regulating task. Most of us do not overperspire year-round, but advertising insists that sweat rings are a constant threat, indoors or out, in hot weather and tepid, and that they are a huge embarrassment. If you have overactive sweat glands, perhaps a steady application of a powerful antiperspirant is necessary. But for most men, heavy perspiration is only an occasional problem. Consider using a normal deodorant most of the time, and the antiperspirant only when you are going to be outside during the hottest days of the year.

LURKING IN THE DARKNESS: Your lower regions also get hot and sticky and could become breeding grounds for smells, bacteria, and rashes. Let's take your front first. Your crotch should be low-maintenance. Good cleaning, rinsing, and drying and a fresh pair of underwear every morning is enough for most guys. Itching and a rash are indicative of allergies or fungal infection. If you are prone to athlete's foot, you may have the crotch version. Over-the-counter ointments or jock-itch sprays and powders that contain miconazole or clortrimazole may be strong enough to kick it in less than a month. If not, get it checked out with a physician or a dermatologist, especially if you could pass it on to a partner.

YOUR PENIS: Keep your friendly member carefully cleaned, and pay special attention under your foreskin if you are not circumcised. Odd discharges, painful urination, or blood in your semen demands professional attention. Don't ignore these symptoms (see appendix, pages 151, 157).

TROUBLE FROM BEHIND: Your rear requires some more thorough attention, particularly if you suffer from itching, hemorrhoids, or constipation. Most itching trouble comes from not cleaning thoroughly after each bowel movement. But don't scrub either, because that can trigger more sensitivity. If irritation is becoming a problem, try using baby wipes lightly after each bowel movement. Then apply a zinc ointment, or even a little Vaseline. Be diligent, and it will probably stop bothering you. See a doctor if you suspect more serious irritation.

If you find comfort in numbers, hemorrhoids—actually enlarged varicose veins—are far more common than you think. Straining on the toilet from constipation is the leading cause of hemorrhoids, and can be eased by a diet high in fiber, grains, fruits, and vegetables and low in dairy products. Drinking lots of water will irrigate and soften your stools. It's a good idea, in fact, to drink two or three glasses of water as soon as you get up in the morning to get your system off to a good, clean start. Coffee doesn't count. Juice does, but drink the water in addition to the juice to be certain your system stays lubed.

PASSING GAS: Gas is produced as your body digests various foods. Some foods—beans are the most common—produce lots of gas, although thorough cooking can reduce that problem. A sudden addition of lots of fruit to your diet can create a similar effect. So too can other high-fiber and fatty foods. In the antacid section of the drugstore, you can find remedies to try if the problem becomes painful or embarrassing.

HEART AND SOUL: Learn how to monitor your heart occasionally for signs of potential trouble. Genetics, the single biggest factor in predicting heart problems, is out of your control, but it is possible to compensate if your family is prone to heart attacks or strokes. The three factors to watch are blood pressure, pulse, and cholesterol levels. Each time you have a physical, get the results of the tests your doctor performs and review them. The medical appendix in the back of the book (see pages 152–53) will help you understand what some of these numbers mean.

PLUMBING PROBLEMS: Maalox is not a health beverage. For men with a stainless steel constitution, plumbing problems mean nothing, but for many men, indigestion, gas, ulcers, and regularity are constant reminders of the stresses they suffer. For too long, stomach distress has been a peculiar badge of male success. In the 1960s it seemed that no truly successful businessman *didn't* have an ulcer. Now doctors know that ulcers are caused by an overuse of aspirin or ibuprofen, by smoking, or by bacterial infection, not by ambition. Better diet, more exercise, and a little perspective on your professional situation can usually calm a raging gut better than an antacid.

COLON AND PROSTATE CANCER are two vital backside concerns. See the early warning signs (page 151) for more on this. You cannot identify colon cancer early yourself; that requires a professionally analyzed stool sample. Prostate problems may be signaled by frequent or painful nighttime urination. These are usually a sign of age rather than

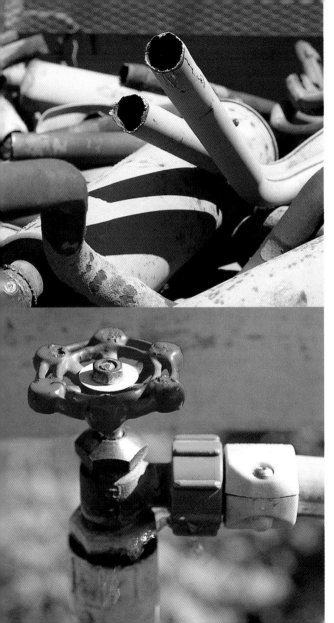

cancer, but get any plumbing problems diagnosed. And even if you don't experience common symptoms, have yourself checked thoroughly and regularly—at least every two or three years—especially after you reach your mid- to late forties.

TESTICULAR CANCER can be self-detected, most easily after a warm shower or bath. Feel for unusual bumps at least once a month and have them checked out immediately. This form of cancer is most common in young men, but can be readily treated if detected early.

SEXUAL DISEASES are deadly serious business, both for yourself and for your sexual partners. Gone are the days when a relatively harmless case of crabs was a teenage rite of passage. Today, sexual viruses, bacteria, parasites, and fungus infections come in new and frightening forms, and there is nothing harmless about any of them. Don't catch or spread them (see pages 156–57). Can this be any simpler?

It's hard to believe that many men (and women) still refuse to practice safe sex with their partners, but statistics prove the point. If you are fooling around, understand the reproductive and medical risks and the implications of what you are doing. Physics make prophylactics effective, so use them properly. Don't assume a woman should take responsibility for contraception or disease prevention. Assume it is your responsibility—always. Passion is great, but it's even better when you know that you don't have to worry about sexual disease or unwanted pregnancy (see pages 156–57).

If you have ever had sex—with anyone— get tested for HIV. Viruses don't care about promises, trust, honesty, and commitments. Those things you can deal with; infections are immune to talk.

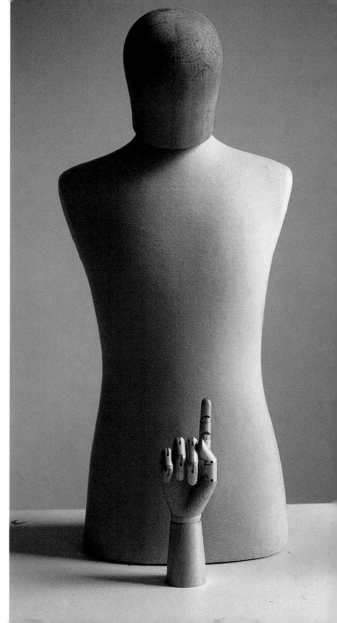

Your Outer Reaches: Hands, Feet, and Nails

HANDS: Many men don't realize how important good hand care is to women. For guys, rough, dry, and callused hands are a badge of the hard physical work they do. In fact, if there were creams to toughen and roughen hands, many guys would use them. But women have a different perspective.

First, keep 'em clean. Have you ever scoffed at some phobic soul who only opens doorknobs with a handkerchief? Perhaps he knows more than you do, or he's seen a demonstration of just how germ-laden door handles—and other people's hands—can be. Statistics that reveal how inconsistently men wash their hands after using the toilet are spooky. The signs in restaurants may be for the employees, but it won't hurt you to follow along. Hot water and soap, used several

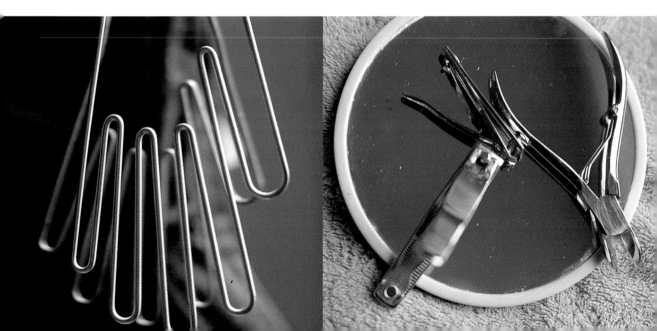

times a day for at least ten full, soapy seconds, will kill many germs and cut down on your chances for catching or passing on colds and other illness. Seriously. Wash your hands. Regularly and often. And even if you do, don't rub your eyes with your fingers.

FINGERNAILS: Keep a nail brush by the sink and use it regularly to keep your nails clean. Beyond that, keep your nails properly trimmed, and they probably won't need any more care than that, unless they are injured or damaged in some way. Then they require quick attention. Treat them well to avoid damaging the skin under your nails. Injured nails are prone to fungal infections that are difficult to eliminate. Like hair, nails can indicate poor nutrition or a more serious health problem, so if you notice that your nails are cracking or brittle, or aren't growing normally, take it as a serious warning sign and discuss it with a doctor or dermatologist. Here are some pointers:

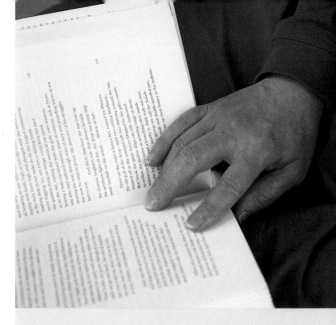

- Don't bite your nails. It is a bad habit that you can't hide.

- Instead of your fangs, use sharp nail clippers or, if you are fussy, nail scissors. Unless you are a hand model or you have exceedingly fast-growing claws, weekly clipping should do it.

- As you trim, follow the profile of your fingertips, and cut just at or below that edge, depending on your preference. Use many small clips instead of one or two big ones.

- Basic nail care is not difficult. As with your beard, your nails trim more cleanly if they have absorbed water. Do it weekly after a shower, while you wait for your shave cream to soften your beard. Some guys make a habit of doing it on a particular day of the week—a Sunday-morning ritual, perhaps.

- Manicures feel great and aren't just for women. If your nails need professional help, have a manicure to get them back in shape so you can resume proper care. Make sure the salon is clean and sterilizes its tools between customers.

- A clear polish? Don't. It's on the wrong side of vanity. Unless you are a hand model, it looks a little too feminine for most guys.

- If you injure your nail enough to split it, or if you get blood under the nail and it is painful and doesn't heal quickly, have a dermatologist check it out. (See toenail care, following.) Remedies include topical prescription creams—which only work in light cases—and systemic medicine, which can cure the fungus, but your kidneys may suffer since they have to filter the medicine out eventually.

TOENAILS: Most of the information about fingernails also applies to your toenails, but since they sit in socks most of the time, take more weight, and are pushed around by your shoes, they are even more prone to pressures and threats, especially fungal infections. And when they are not in socks, they may be padding around gym locker rooms and shower stalls—breeding grounds for the fungus that causes athlete's foot. Nail fungus is an elaboration of the stuff that irritates skin between your

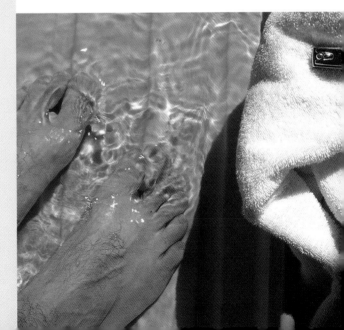

toes, except that it crawls under your toenails. Injured nails are much more prone to fungus than healthy ones, and an established case is difficult to dislodge.

Fungus is characterized by a yellowing of the nail, and eventually a thick, flaky degradation of the tissue. Fortunately, it's not going to go much farther than your nail, but it looks gross, you can infect your sleeping partner, and it's something you'd rather not have. Podiatrists can sometimes treat it by grinding the nail down to the quick, eliminating as much as possible, and covering what is left with a prescription ointment. This may only arrest the fungus,

since it is persistent stuff. Some podiatrists recommend a systemic approach with prescription drugs, but others feel that the potential kidney damage isn't worth the risk for mild cases.

Toenails require heartier clippers with straighter, only slightly convex blades. These prevent you from reaching too far into the corners when you trim. Do not overtrim. Wet nails are more easily trimmed than dry ones, and on your big toenail, take several smaller clips instead of one big one. A pedicure is a princely indulgence, but it can be helpful every blue moon to put your toenails right— if you aren't prohibitively ticklish!

THE REST OF YOUR FEET: As anyone who has survived corrective foot surgery will tell you, it's no fun. Given the complexity of the bones, muscles, ligaments, tendons, and blood that courses through the works, you want to keep your feet happy, all life long.

- Wear good shoes. If any piece of clothing can be considered an investment, it is a good pair of shoes. Fortunately, no one has ever tried to convince guys that wearing four-inch stilettos is a smart fashion idea. Mostly, men can select from a range of sensible shoes.

- A well-made pair of shoes that fits properly is essential to good foot care. The best shoes have firm support. Unlike bedroom slippers, they should feel tighter in the arch. There should be enough room for your toes so they don't bunch, and the back should hold on to the heel as you walk.

- Unless you want them to become rubber petri dishes for fungi and bacteria, dry your gym or running shoes between wearings. If you keep them in a gym locker, rotate pairs. Allow forty-eight hours between wearings if possible.

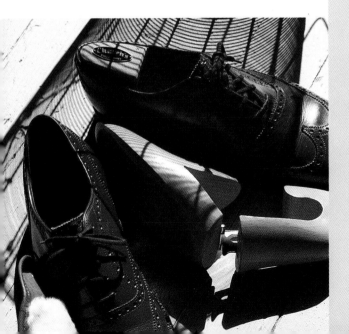

CHAPTER 2

Weight Maintenance

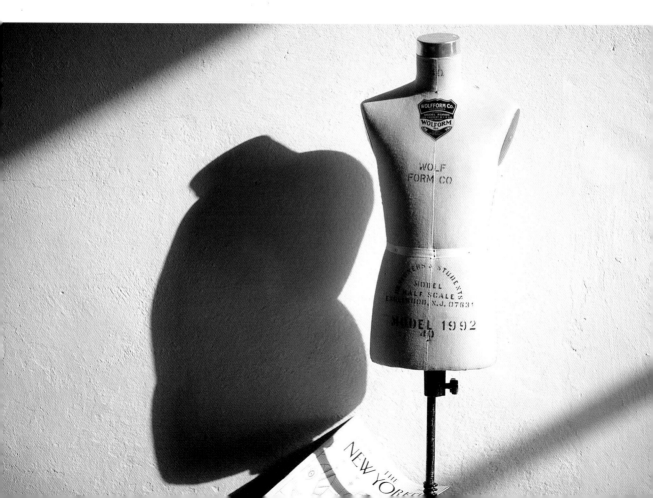

Diet

If anything, there are too many diets and eating routines available today. Many are difficult to understand, require devotion to dietary rites that are hard to maintain, and have gimmicks that may not fit your taste or basic lifestyle. That said, if you are unhappy with your weight, you need to adjust both your exercise routine and your diet.

- Your body needs to take in less fuel and burn up its extra reserves.

- The more muscle you have, the more calories your body will burn all day and all night, with or without exercise.

- If you go on a strict diet without increasing your exercise, you will lose weight, but some of it will be muscle mass, which means your body won't need as many calories to survive, so your metabolism will slow down to accommodate your new eating habits.

- If you exercise more and continue to eat as you did before, you will lose fat, but your weight may not change, as more mass is converted to heavier muscle. Generally, that's okay with most men.

- If you are too fat and want to be stronger and leaner, adjust your diet to include much less fat and sugar, adequate protein, and a good balance of carbohydrates. And exercise a lot, with emphasis on aerobic activity.

- If you want to be stronger and bulkier, adjust your diet to include much more protein and a good balance of carbohydrates. Emphasize weight training.

- The only men who need to increase fat in their diets are those who live in extreme cold and rely on fat to store energy. For most men, that's not the case. Are you eating for an Antarctic winter?

- The back of this book (pages 154–55) has some useful basic caloric formulas to help you figure how you can adjust your intake and exercise levels to shed some pounds and get stronger.

SYSTEM CLEANSING, FASTS, DIETS, HEALTHY JUICES: It may sound appealing to subject yourself to a rigorous fast, and if you are in good health it may not do you any harm, but some simple adjustments to your diet may achieve similar results. A week-long diet without fast food, with lots of fruit, salads, fresh vegetables, healthy grains, hearty breads, and less meat might help your whole digestive tract feel stronger and less touchy. Extend that diet by a week, and you may discover that you prefer eating that way. Try making this general dietary approach the norm rather than the exception, and much of your excess weight may disappear as a result.

The amount of salt used in processed and restaurant-prepared foods is staggering. Its only purpose is to enhance taste, but your blood pressure suffers the consequences. Look at it this way: restaurants—high-, low-, and medium-grade—want their food to be memorable, so they enhance basic flavors with salt. Many take it even farther by adding a little sugar to contrast with the salt. Food processors who create canned, frozen, and other packaged meals do the same. They want their products to register in your memory so you will buy them again.

After years of this bombardment of oversalted foods, our taste buds come to expect those sensations, and register disappointment when they don't get a buzz. But salt masks the true taste of food. We lose our ability to pick out and enjoy more subtle tastes and seasonings. One of the best ways to diet is to prepare as many meals as you can yourself—or order your meals in restaurants with much more care. Order meals with the most natural ingredients in their most unprocessed states. Stay away from creamy sauces. Order salads with dressing on the side, and use it sparingly.

Fresh fruit and vegetable juices, ones you prepare or order from a juice bar, can be great meals in themselves. A lunch of a fruit or vegetable drink and a plain tortilla or whole wheat bagel can be a delicious and satisfying meal, low in salt and fat. Here are two simple recipes you can make in a blender, but feel free to experiment.

Tomato, Parsley, Bell Pepper Juice

2 ripe medium to large tomatoes
1 cup (15 g) loosely packed parsley with stems
1 red or yellow bell pepper, seeded with stem
    removed

Process in a blender by starting with one tomato;
then add the parsley. When thoroughly blended,
add the pepper, then the second tomato.
Makes one large serving.

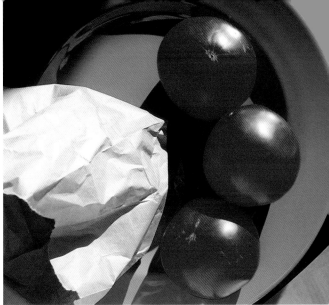

Plum, Peach, Blueberry Smoothie

3 plums, pitted
1 peach, peeled and pitted
1 cup (140 g) blueberries
½ cup (120 ml) milk, yogurt, or ice-cream, as desired

Blend to desired consistency.
Makes one medium serving.

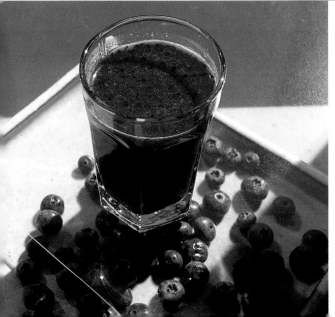

CHANGING YOUR RELATIONSHIP TO FOOD: The percentage of overweight people in America grows every year, and it's not healthy. There are many factors: stress and emotional problems that encourage unhealthy eating patterns, a lack of vigorous exercise, easy access to absurdly fatty fast food, and bad dietary habits that become ingrained patterns.

A healthier approach is to reevaluate your relationship to food. Is your stomach leading you around from one unnecessary snack to another? Does your gut have to tighten a little to feel as if it has had a proper meal? And do you eat so quickly that you don't feel your stomach tighten until it is too late, and then you feel stuffed? No one likes to be bullied, but perhaps that's what your appetite is doing to you. With the right attitude, you can adjust those habits and take control of them. Chapter 4 offers suggestions for reducing stress, which often triggers overeating.

THE FRENCH APPROACH: You can also take the advice of Julia Child, who admonishes us to eat well, but in moderation. Easy to say, but harder to put into regular practice. The way the French see it, most Americans don't taste, we swallow; taste becomes a drive-by sensation. The French also teach children in elementary school about qualities and distinctions in tastes. French children learn that a spoonful portion, savored and tasted lingeringly, can be far more satisfying and just as filling as a whole cupful of the same dish gulped down like dog food. This important part of their culture and heritage—this sensitivity to subtle taste distinctions—is a source of enormous pride to the French. Their eating habits also discourage between-meal snacks and constant grazing; meals are for mealtime, and that's that. Despite the abundance of cream, butter, meats, and other high-fat ingredients in the national diet, obesity is not a serious problem in France. So perhaps the best way to change your caloric intake is to change your relationship to your food. You may find that in doing so, you not only eat less but enjoy it more.

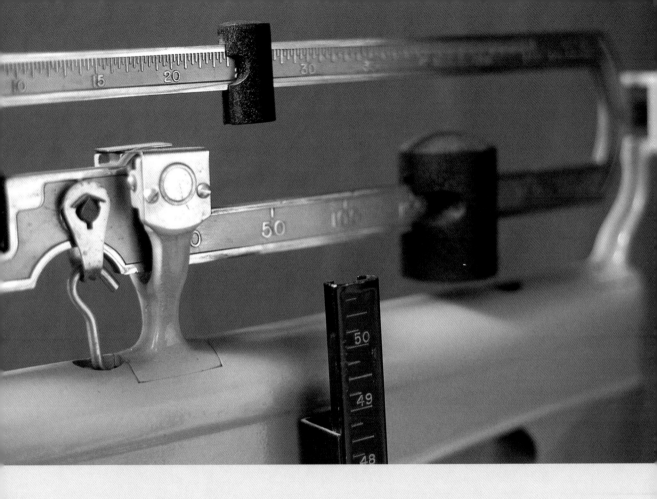

Fitness

Every man would like to be fitter than he is. Stronger, more coordinated, quicker on his feet. Some goals are realistic, and others are frustrating fantasies. You can and should, however, become generally fit. You may not ever win the swimsuit competition or Iron Man Triathlon, but you should be able to bound up a few flights of stairs without wheezing, or even go out on a day-long hike without a respirator. As an act of male responsibility to your family, friends, and loved ones, stay reasonably fit. If you are not now, start gradually and work at it steadily. Sooner than you might imagine, your clothes will feel better, your posture will improve, and your self-image will get the boost it needs.

WORKING OUT ONE DAY AT A TIME: Regular, sensible exercise is far better than occasional heroic starts and stops. Ever noticed how much more crowded the gym is right after New Year's than even a month later? That's how fleeting good fitness intentions are. Most fitness experts will tell you that it is because most of us try to take on too much, our goals are unrealistic, and we don't have the time or the willpower (and perhaps even the genetic disposition) to become a specimen of buffed muscle. Discouragement sets in, and the negative cycle resumes.

These same fitness experts will also tell you that a little exercise several times a week, in regular half-hour sessions that don't overtax your schedule, your system, or your dedication, will in the end make you healthier and stronger. It's the regular, healthy fitness patterns that eventually build into successful fitness routines. And as the pattern grows stronger, and it is easier to work out regularly, you may find it easier to toughen your routine and to push yourself harder. If you are diligent, you will end up with a fitter body than you ever imagined.

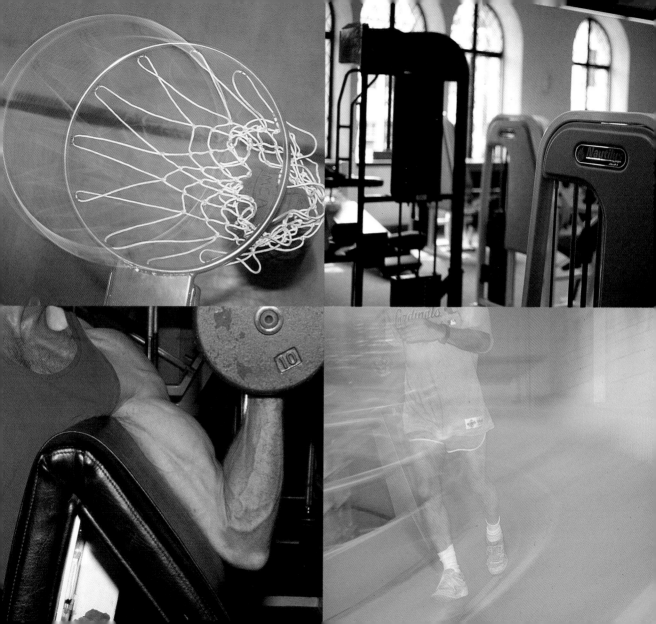

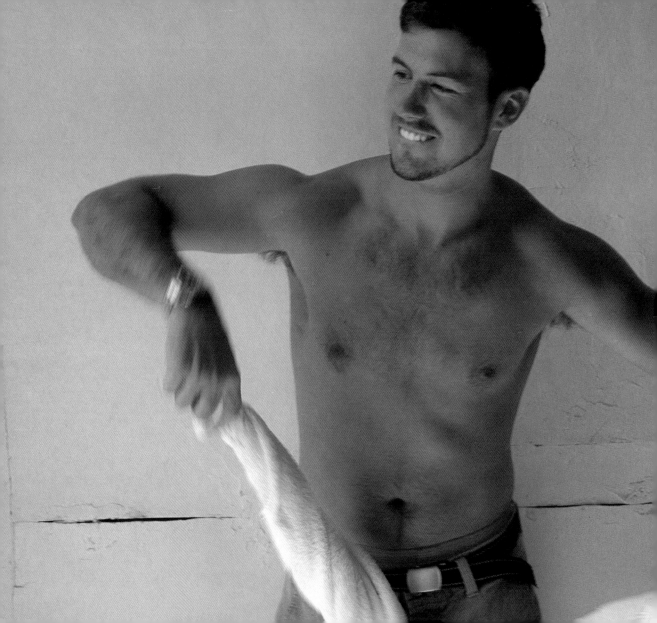

Finding the right time of day to exercise is an obstacle for many working men. Some exercise routines encourage morning workouts to increase metabolic activity throughout the day. Mornings can also be efficient because you can combine your morning and workout showers to save time. But many men find that lunch-time works better because it is easier to eat lighter after a workout. For others, the end of the day beats them all. It's a terrific mental refresher. Ironically, working out earlier in the day may increase your late-day energy, and working out too late can make sleep more difficult. Regardless of when a workout works best for you, make it a routine.

PICKING A ROUTINE AND A GYM:
Pick a variety of activities you enjoy doing so you don't get bored. You may enjoy the treadmill, but give the rowing machine a regular workout too, to make sure you are toning all parts of your body. If swimming comes most easily to you, give the stair machines a try. Cross training is an excellent tool, so remember to use it.

Find a gym you actually look forward to visiting. Some men find weight lifters and body-builders intimidating to be around; others find them inspiring. Some find gyms in office towers too homogeneous and enjoy a mix of ages, backgrounds, economic levels, and fitness levels. In most cities gyms now come in many styles, so shop around and pick one that fits your disposition and your schedule.

BASIC STRETCHES AND WARM-UPS:

Professional athletes warm up. You should too. For muscles, nerves, connective tissue, joints, reflexes, and your mind to be working properly, the body needs all of its systems engaged and in sync. Although you would benefit from twenty minutes of stretching each workout, most guys are pressed for time, so warm up efficiently. A brisk, ten-minute walk to the gym will get things moving and ready for your basketball game. Or if you are using weight machines, even a few minutes of stretches will help. Then, starting gently, let the activity on the first machine warm you up for the second, and so on. A session of sit-ups can be a good way to get much of the body all in gear, and it's generally a good idea to get tougher exercises like ab work out of the way early when you have the most energy. Stretching not only helps specific muscles remain well circulated and limber but encourages you to perform a quick systems check. A stretch can reveal how much tension you are holding. The following can and should be done during your workday, as well as at the gym.

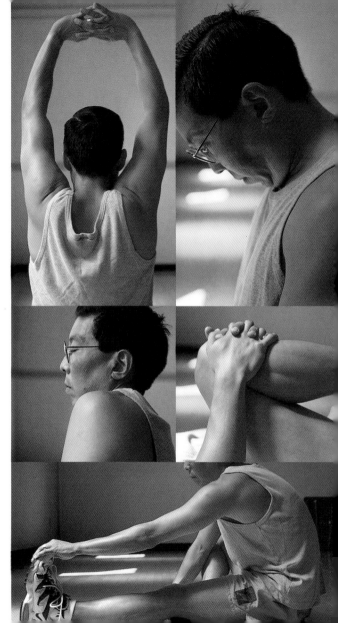

Five Easy Stretches

- Back, torso, shoulders, arms: Standing, mesh your fingers together and reach as high as you can, palms facing up. Lift yourself as high as you can, so you feel the stretch from your thighs and abs, into your chest, shoulders, and arms. Hold the stretch for 20 seconds to 1 minute. Slowly stretch at the waist from right to left to get extra benefit.

- Neck and shoulders: For most men, stress sits on their neck and shoulders. Whether you lift weights, shovel coal, or sit at a computer terminal all day, you will end up with a stiff neck if you don't give it a good stretch many times throughout the day. Once started, a stiff neck is difficult to shake. At your desk, or standing, simply hang your head forward, letting its weight stretch the muscles along the back, central shoulders, and down toward the spine; this will make the entire area much less tense. You can also lower both shoulders and move your head to one side so your ear tries to touch the lowered shoulder. (Unless you are a contortionist, this won't be possible.) Then slowly and gently pivot your head down so your chin and jaw roll against your collarbones until you can let your other ear try to pull toward its lowered shoulder. Do not rock your head backward toward your spine; this can cause injury.

- Another good neck and shoulder stretch: Pull your shoulders up to your ears and rotate the shoulders in a circular motion as though you were swimming the breaststroke. Go forward for a minute or two, and then reverse direction. Slow, deliberate, and thorough stretches will do more good than quick bunny motions.

- Back: Lying on your back, pull one knee up to your chest. Pull gently on your knee to feel the stretch. Hold for 20 seconds. Lower the leg and repeat with your other leg.

- Hamstrings: Sitting on the floor, straighten one leg and put the sole of the other foot against the inside of your thigh. Reach to your toes and pull them toward you slightly. Gently bend forward until you feel the stretch in the back of your straightened thigh. Hold for at least 20 seconds. Switch legs and repeat.

AEROBIC AND WEIGHT TRAINING:

It's now well known that you need both aerobic and weight training to keep your entire system at its peak. Cardiovascular benefits of aerobic exercise are clear, but more doctors are realizing that weight training builds and retains muscle tissue and is essential for building and preserving bone tissue. Even elderly men should continue to lift weights to reduce bone loss and damage from injury.

Finding the right balance between the two kinds of exercise is important. If you want to bulk up and increase the size of your muscle mass, you will need a specific workout routine of high weights/low reps to achieve that. If you prefer a strong, tough, leaner look, you will want a routine with many repetitions of more manageable weight and lots of aerobic activity to burn off the extra fat you are carrying. In any case, steady, routine devotion is all-important.

THE PAIN OF GAIN:

Heavy exercise, particularly weight lifting, breaks down the muscle tissue. As it is built back up, it grows in size and strength. Muscular aches from working muscles that haven't been used for a while are caused by buildups of metabolic wastes that take time to wash out of your system. This process is necessary, although if your stiffness is debilitating, you have worked too hard, too quickly. Take it easy. Slower development with less weight is better for building up strength in your joints too.

If you are trying to build muscle mass, you shouldn't lift weights each day with the same set of muscles: the body needs forty-eight hours to rebuild new muscle tissue. Working those muscle sets every day may actually make them smaller and tighter. You can, however, work on your upper body one day and lower body the next, and so on, but you may want to cross-train instead, with an aerobic day to keep your activities in balance.

RECOVERY TIME: Even if you are doing daily aerobics in an effort to lose extra fat, alternate your activities. For example, if you run on Monday and want an aerobic exercise for Tuesday, try swimming, the rowing machine, or some other low-impact aerobic activity so your knees and foot joints can adjust to Monday's effort. Although you can find good old troopers who run each day, for every one of them there are many others who can no longer run at all because they overdid it.

Treat muscular aches with ice packs for serious muscle strain and minor injuries, and heat for simple relaxation. Long, hot baths help, as does stretching. In fact, if you finish a workout or a long run and you think some muscular pain is up ahead, do a slow series of stretches, for at least twenty minutes, stretching the muscles you have overused and holding them stretched for at least thirty seconds to a minute. You will be surprised how much that can reduce muscular aches the next day.

The actual, physical value of lineament rubs is questionable, but the psychological benefit of the smell of menthol makes them aces. For something a little more exotic than the usual menthol rub, try Tiger Balm. It is probably the single most popular medicine in much of Asia, and the warm, soothing smells of clove and camphor and penetrating radiance of menthol make this a hit hard to resist. Combine the rub with a massage, which heals by increasing circulation, forcing blood through all of the muscle fibers. Massage also helps uric acid buildup move out of the muscle tissue.

SIMPLE SPORTS INJURIES: Injuries—cuts, scrapes, bruises, and sprains—are painful, and the older you are, the more care and attention you need to give them. Age raises the stakes.

- When you were a boy, your mom probably took care of most cuts and scrapes with soap, water, and peroxide, or some other disinfectant. You are a big boy now, but it is just as important to clean and treat each injury. Adults are still prone to infection, and adult skin doesn't heal as quickly as it once did.

- Sprains, pulled muscles, torn muscles, joint trouble, and other common injuries also need appropriate care. An ice pack is less appealing than a hot bath, but more effective at reducing swelling.

- Each injury requires its own treatment, but be smart about how quickly you deal with it and how long recovery will take. Repeated injuries to the same part expand and intensify the damage. Learn to heal properly.

- Accidents happen, but self-inflicted injuries may be avoided by warming up properly, playing smart, watching where you are going, and keeping your enthusiastic adrenal rushes in check.

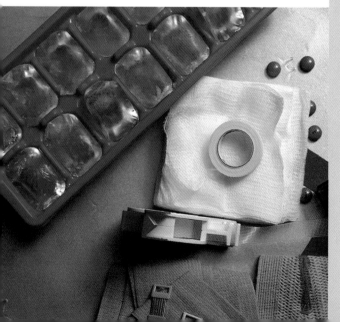

CHAPTER 3

Wardrobe Basics

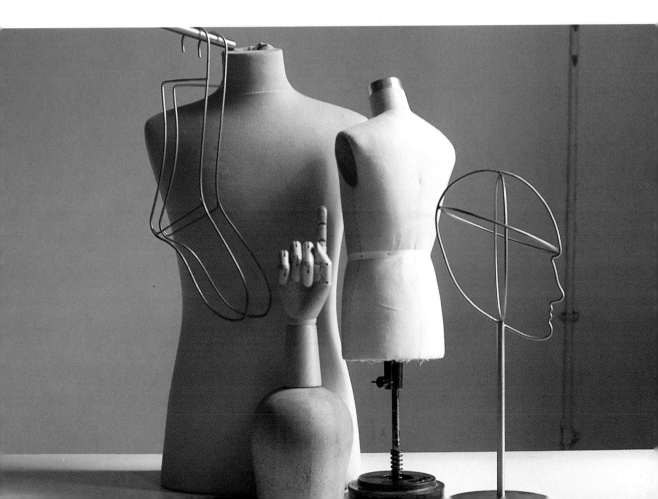

Clothes You Could Wear
for the Rest of Your Life

Women, in general, build a fashion whole from many pieces. If you have the money, time, and talent, you can become a full-fledged clotheshorse, and for some men in some professions, it's even expected. But most of us aren't, and that's what makes dressing so simple for men. We can look great with a few standard items of good quality that fit well and are flattering. With a few accessories—ties being the most common—we can spruce up those basic items with a little more polish. Or not. That's the beauty—men can get away with a basic, practical, and handsome set of uniforms and look great! So take advantage of this.

Ralph Lauren proved in his ads that you can look terrific in a blazer, a blue cotton work shirt, and a pair of worn jeans. Although to be fair, Ralph is rarely in an office setting in those photos, so you will probably need a few more items. But not many. Make sure you have the basics covered first.

Studies have consistently shown that women are more attuned than men to clothes their peers are wearing; take a lesson from them, and notice the clothes of friends, men you work with, or guys you pass on the street. Observe general "looks"—combinations of jackets, shirts, ties, slacks, and shoes. Notice what good-looking men of comparable builds, age, coloring, and profession wear well. Chances are, they are wearing some classic basics. Recreational and underclothes aside, you could make a short list of clothes that would serve you well to your grave. They would probably need to be replaced occasionally, but let's see just how simple it can be.

THE BLAZER: Nothing is more versatile and good looking than a well-cut, well-made navy blue wool blazer. Unless you live in the tropics, you'll need one in felt wool for winter and one in serge wool for the summer. Try on many from different stores before buying one; you will know when you've found the right one for you by the way it fits and looks. A blazer is more versatile without the gold buttons; if the blazer of your dreams has them, have the buttons replaced with dark ones, or go live on a boat. Single vents are most practical and versatile.

THE SPORT JACKET: Sport jackets come in many colors, types of cloths, and cuts. Buy a navy blazer first, but if you want more variety a nice wool, silk and wool, or linen sport jacket is a good investment. If you like a pattern, make it subtle. As for cut, make it classic single vent with medium-width lapels if you plan to keep it for more than five years.

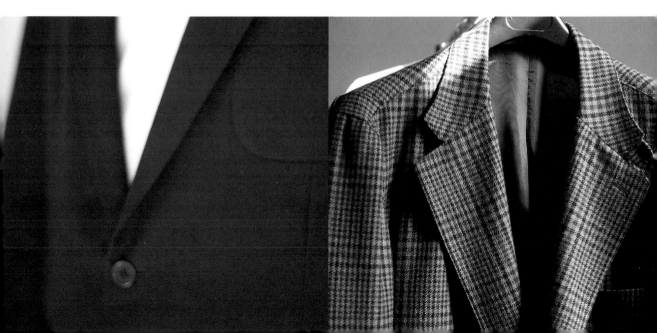

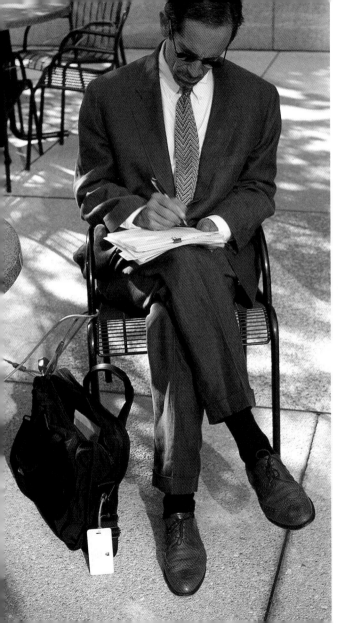

THE SUIT: In many offices the look is strictly casual all week, not just on Fridays. But even if you are fresh out of college, you need a suit. If you only have one, make it a good, conservative but comfortably cut model, in a medium-weight wool. Gray is the most versatile, but navy is a good second choice. (You can wear the gray slacks with your navy blazer too, but navy slacks with the navy blazer is a mistake.) If you work in an office that expects more formal attire, you should add more suits in a variety of styles—but start with the gray.

How many suits do you need? Unless you are flat broke, buy enough suits to allow you to rotate them. Clothes last much longer if you give them at least a day or two to air out and dry, and of course, to go to the cleaners.

SLACKS, CHINOS, AND JEANS: Again, you can't beat the classics. Gray flannel in two seasonal weights will serve you well. Since you wear your pants all day, and probably take your jacket off for most of it, consider buying two pairs of slacks for each blazer. Some men who have their suits tailored, in fact, regularly order a double pair for their workhorse suits.

Chinos. Ah, chinos, also known as khakis for their most common color—all cotton, comfortable, relatively cheap, easy to clean, lots of sizes to choose from, in safe, conservative colors. You can never have too many, but make sure they fit. Given the countless size, color, brand, and style variations available today, you have no excuse if you can't find a pair that flatter your body.

And everyone's favorite, jeans. It should be easier to look good in jeans than most men do. But men often don't look very good in jeans for some basic reasons: they are the wrong size, they are the wrong cut, or they are worn with tops that make them look cheap and sloppy. Jeans look great when they are contrasted with something special. A pair of jeans with a good pair of leather shoes and a clean, white, pressed oxford shirt to set them off. Or another American classic, jeans and a T-shirt (see pages 12–17 for T-shirt fit), perhaps with a pair of tennis shoes. The T-shirt should be really clean and very white without any logo emblazoned on it—a classic look should not turn you into a billboard. Black jeans can create a slightly more formal look than classic blue. For other colors, stick to chinos.

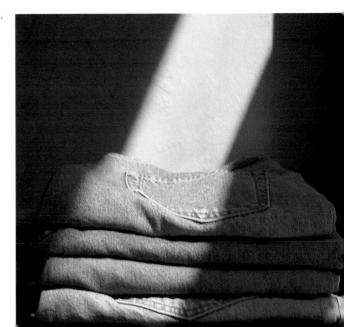

SHIRTS: Polo shirts are always smart, but knits do reveal the general contours of the body. So long as you are trim enough, wear them. Otherwise, stick to button-down shirts, which drape better. Stay with solids, and you can wear strong colors without looking goofy. Stripes and funny patterns should be reserved for the golf course.

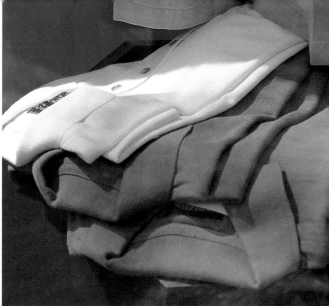

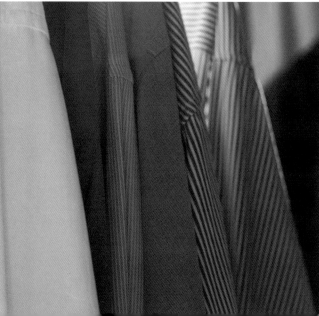

Dress shirts don't need to be any more complicated than good-quality cotton, in white, off-white, and blue. Oxford cloth is durable and ages well. Finer cottons feel great, but they are more vulnerable to stains and signs of wear. Classic collars should be selected to suit your face shape. Button-down collars are slightly less formal and go better with the blazer than the suit—although it is no crime to wear them together during the business day. Wear a regular collar with a suit at a more formal dinner.

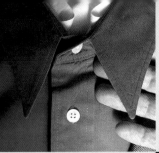

Classic collars can be worn with or without ties. Fasten the top button.

Classic collars with longer points are best for normal to round faces. Shorter points are best for normal to long faces.

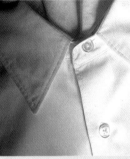

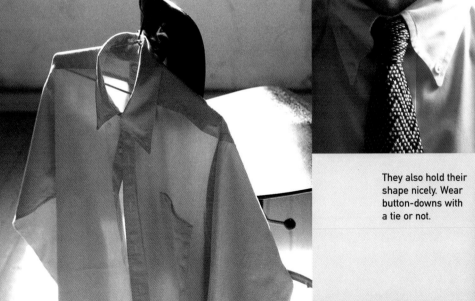

Button-downs are preppier than classic collars.

They also hold their shape nicely. Wear button-downs with a tie or not.

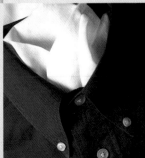

SWEATERS: Light wool or cotton sweaters in the summer. Heavier wool in the winter. Keep them simple, not too tight, in darker colors. Fold them carefully after each use—no hangers. Sweaters are classic and easy; it's hard to go wrong.

TIES: For many men, buying ties might as well be rocket science, but you can't go wrong when you follow these pointers:

- A guy can get away with five to ten ties, if the variety is wide enough, if they suit the clothes they are worn with, and if they are handsome enough.

- Buy silk ties, although cotton ties can work in the summer—on the hottest days.

- The more subtle the pattern and color, the longer you can wear a tie.

- Ties with black, brown, and other dark colors are more versatile because they can be worn with black or brown shoes.

- Learn to tie a tie carefully and properly.

- Wear your ties at the right length. The point should not extend beyond your belt.

- Thick ties make big, fat knots, so beware.

- Properly selected and cared for, ties will last several years (see page 90).

- In the morning, choose a tie based on the clothes you are wearing it with. If you are wearing a gray suit, black shoes and belt, and a white or blue shirt, select one that has a deep color, with at least a little blue, and a black field or background in the pattern. Don't select a pale gray. A brown jacket will work better with a tie that has some browns or neutral tones in the background, but the primary color should provide a solid contrast to the jacket fabric.

- Don't buy goofball ties unless you have the personality and *chutzpah* to pull it off.

- Bow ties can and do work on some men. Try one if you are tempted, but make sure it is a tied one and not a clip-on.

Tying a Tie

{FOUR IN HAND}

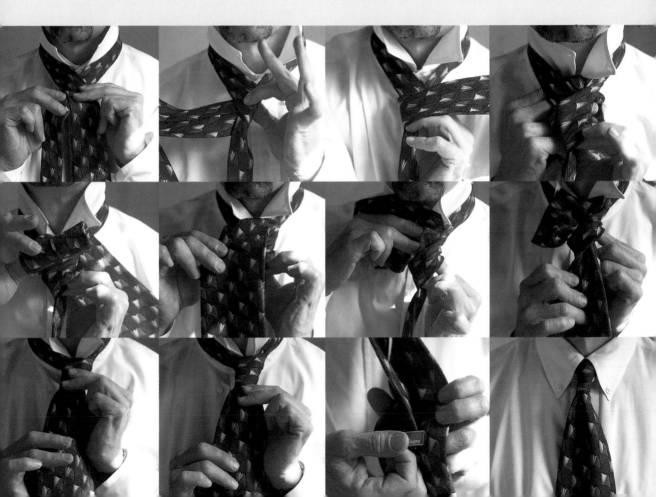

SHOES: Shoes give a guy away, so go for quality. Athletic shoes are fine in the gym, but it is hard to imagine classic men—say Cary Grant or Gary Cooper—bounding around in them. Sure, times have changed, but if you are old enough to buy a drink, you are old enough to wear good shoes. Yes, even when you aren't at work. Get used to it.

Shoes are expensive. As with most clothes, shoes need to rest between wearings, so invest in four or five pairs to get you started. You need a black pair, a dark brown or oxblood pair, and nicer casual shoes that fit your activities and climate. Wear loafers in the city; boots in the rougher country. Deck shoes are nice classics, as are good-quality suede oxfords. Watch for shoe sales, and you can save a bundle. A good pair of shoes can run over $200, but half-price sales at the end of a season can allow you to double your daily shoe options quickly.

If you really can't afford to invest in expensive shoes, there are some handsome alternatives. Look for the most conservative, simplest knockoffs of the real thing. Make sure they really fit before you buy them. Cut off any labels or tags the manufacturer may have sewn into a seam. They can pass until you can afford the higher grades.

To maintain your good leather shoes, wear them no more frequently than every other day. You will have them around for several years longer if you keep cedar shoe trees inside them when they are not in use. The wood soaks up perspiration, keeps the leather from molding, and maintains their proper shape and profile. Well-made soles, whether leather or rubber, can be replaced as they age, and if you maintain the tops with regular polishing, you'll get many, many fine miles out of them.

Belts should match your shoes in color and texture. Replace them before they look as if they pulled a Calistoga wagon across the prairie.

JEWELRY: Generally, less is more, and a little is way too much.

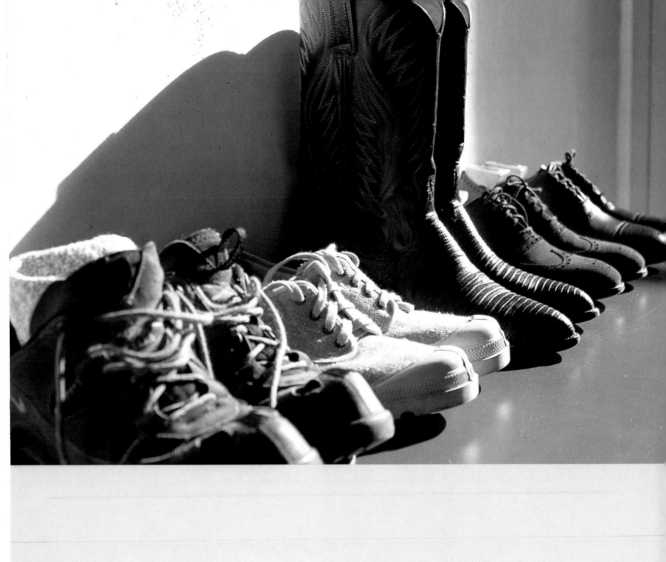

Wear this pair of slacks shopping—when you aren't tired or hungry—so you have a good example to show to the salesperson, or as your own reality check. Keep these points in mind:

- There are many brands of slacks. Promise yourself not to buy any until you have tried on at least five brands, cuts, and sizes.

- Check the size carefully. Are they comfortable? Are they as comfortable as the slacks you wore in to the store?

- Read the laundering instructions carefully to make sure you know how to clean them. If they can be washed, will they shrink? Will you remember to ask your laundry to dry-clean them if you don't want them to shrink?

- Will they go with your jackets?

- Will you wear them?

- If you have cuffs put in slacks, make sure you are wearing them with the waist at the proper height, not too low. Shorter men usually should not wear pants with cuffs.

Once you've found slacks that work, buy and wear them several times. Do these have potential to replace your favorites? If so, go back and buy a few more pairs. If not, continue your search. One secret to shopping simple is to stick with what works for you, and if you can solve the slacks problem, the other items on your list will be a cinch.

SETTING STANDARDS: Men don't need twelve varieties of socks. Black socks go with almost everything. Once a year, go to the store and buy ten pairs of black socks, same brand, same style. Then you never have to worry about matching them up, losing them in the laundry, or trying to figure out if the colors or style are going to look right that day. Although black socks are appropriate with all business attire, you may want to add a few pair of brown socks to go with chinos or brown slacks.

If you have found a great white dress shirt with a collar style that looks good open at the neck or with your ties, with sleeves that are the right length, and in a material that holds up to repeated launderings, buy several at once and rotate them. You may not have to worry about shopping for shirts for a year or more.

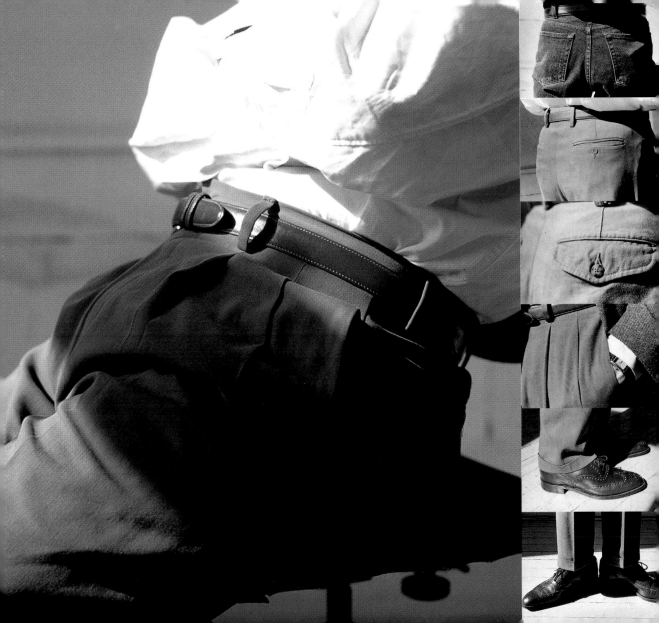

What to Wear When

This is a topic that can make women crazy. As simple as the rules are for men, many get it wrong. When in doubt, dress a little better than you think you need to, because it is always better to be slightly overdressed than underdressed. If you are calling on a new client, wear a suit and tie. A dinner invitation? Same advice. A cocktail party after work? Same. A barbecue? You can lose the tie, but wear sharper clothes than you would hauling stuff to the dump.

Watch out for the word "casual"; in some circles that still means a nice sports jacket and slacks and better shoes. If you really don't know, it never hurts to ask your host or someone else who is attending.

Formal dress means a suit and tie, and in the evening darker is better. If the invitation clearly states black tie, that is what is expected, so you should rent one. (If you go to more than two or three a year, invest in a classic tux. It will fit and look better than a rented one, and you will eventually recoup the cost.) If the black-tie event is sprung on you too late to arrange for one—and if you are not the focus of the event—you can probably sneak by with a very, very dark suit, but a tweed jacket just won't pass.

Casual Fridays have become the norm in most offices. Use the typical dress as the standard and dress down *slightly* from there if you want to. In some settings, jeans are never appropriate; in others they are de rigueur. When in doubt, dress better than your adolescent side hopes it can get away with.

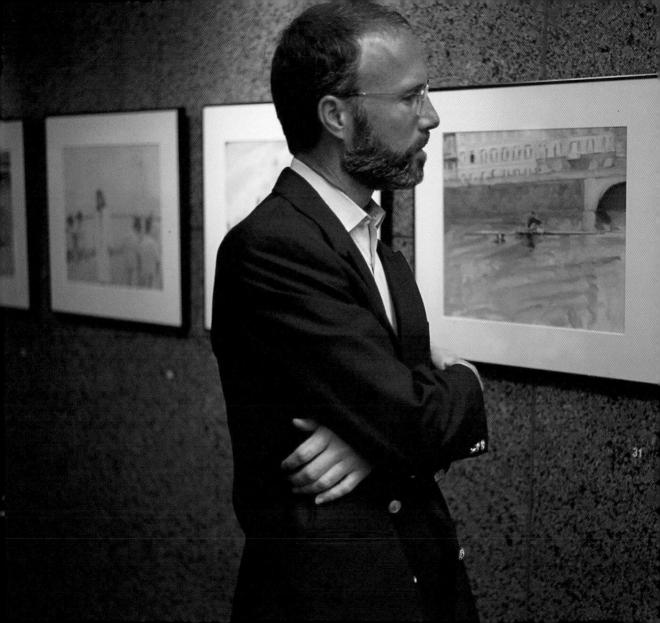

Wash or Dry:
Tips for Clothes Care

If you are sold on the idea that the clothes you are buying are an investment, take care of them as though they are. Follow instructions on the label and you can't go wrong.

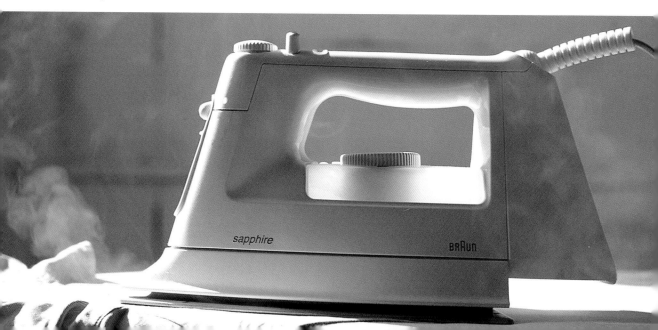

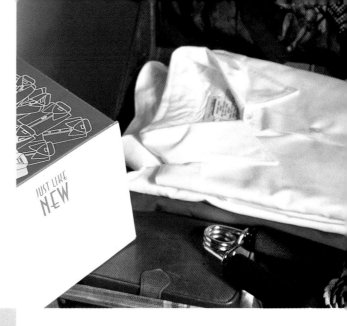

JUST LIKE NEW

LEARN TO DO YOUR OWN LAUNDRY: Unless you send your clothes out to a laundry, learn to wash your clothes properly. If Mom never taught you, it's never too late for a lesson. The rules are simple:

- Read care labels and follow their instructions.

- Wash darks and lights separately, and never wash dark colors in hot water.

- Rinse stains right after you notice them. Letting them sit allows them to set, and makes them harder to remove.

- Soak stains with a stain remover before washing.

- Don't use hotter water than necessary.

- Use detergent sparingly.

- Don't overload the washer or dryer.

LEARN TO IRON YOUR OWN SHIRTS: They will last twice as long. It's true.

TAKEN TO THE CLEANERS: Repeated dry cleaning is rough on clothes, and it changes the texture of most fabric. When a suit has been worn to a smoky lounge, or has soaked up too much body odor, dry clean it. But minor spills should be cleaned up immediately with a damp cloth. Brushing your garments can also keep them cleaner. Pressing is just that.

TIED UP: Silk ties rarely dry-clean well. You are much better off treating these expensive items gingerly:

- Tie them properly (see pages 78–79).

- The most damage is done untying a necktie, so remove it gently and slowly, undoing the knot in the reverse order you tied it to prevent stretching. Don't yank.

- If you spot or stain it with food or drink, immediately dab it with a little water to dilute the stain, and then take the tail end of your tie—the part that doesn't show when you are wearing it—and gently rub the wet spot. The dry silk will help absorb the moisture as it softens the edge of the stain. This helps reduce water spotting. Have the spot removed by a dry cleaner when necessary.

A GOOD SHINE: All shoes should be kept up. A quick professional polish is money well spent; it protects the shoes and keeps them looking good. If you are so inclined, buy a shoeshine kit and keep them up that way.

IN THE CLOSET: Twice each year, with the passing of winter to summer and summer to winter, go through your closet and get rid of anything you know you will never wear. Then pull out all the clothes for storage. Make sure they are clean—moths attack food stains first. (It's not the wool, it's the pasta sauce you left on your lapel that they like.) Put them away with mothballs, cedar chips, or other pest repellents or, if you are lucky enough to have them, in cedar closets or chests. Don't pack them too tightly, and leave them out of their plastic cleaner bags. Cloth needs some ventilation.

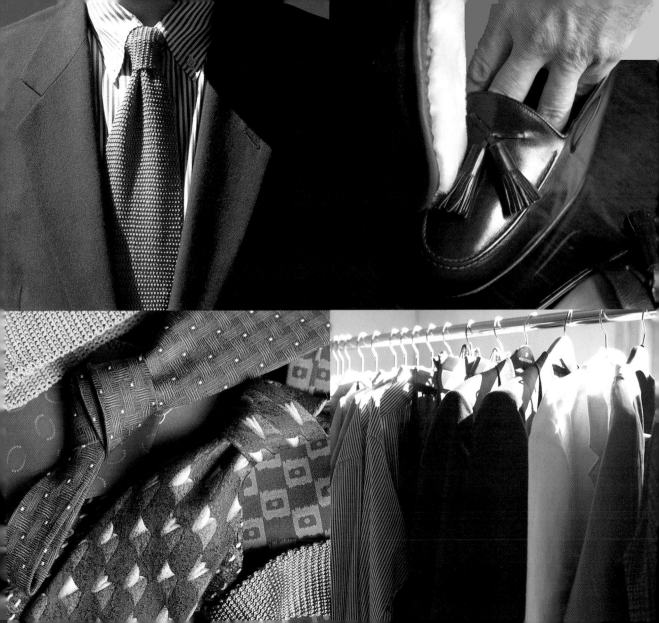

CHAPTER 4

Recharge Your Life

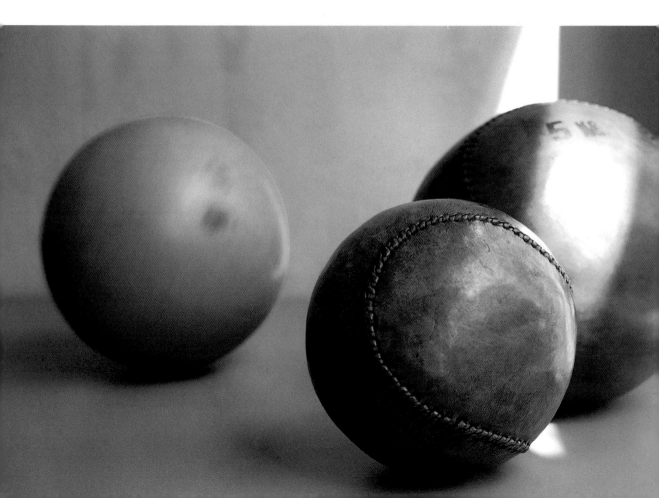

In a perfect world, you would have a terrific job that would only take a few hours a day so you could spend the rest of the time with your family and friends, developing a great physique, improving your mind (or your golf game), and leading a life of excitement and occasional adventure. Your reality probably falls somewhat short of that, especially if you have to work hard for a living and have important commitments and responsibilities.

When everything is going well, you know how good it feels to succeed, to have unlimited energy, to be at the top of your game. But lows come too. If they are occasional and short-lived they are no big deal, but if they are frequent and last longer, they will start stacking up, and you'll lose your charge. Your daily life—and spirit—will start to suffer. In extreme cases you—or your fist—may hit the wall.

Instead of getting caught in a bad cycle, making frequent mistakes or decisions that complicate your life and leave you even more stressed than before, concentrate on things that you enjoy and that will show positive results. This chapter outlines ways you can take control over your body, your attitude, and yourself. Using simple techniques, you can tune up your body and your life to restore it to what it once was or to what you want it to become.

Stress is a given, so work with it. Recognize it for what it is, and redirect it with a change in routine, exercise, relaxation, or a combination of all three. Some stress you choose—accepting a major assignment or a promotion, for example. Other stress is beyond your control or choice— dealing with sick or elderly loved ones, getting laid off from work, an accident, or other misfortunes. These sad things are a part of life and you still need to deal with them. Staying on top of it, managing stress as best you can, helps you maintain a more rational balance.

The Big Picture

Stress works like this:

- Stress motivates in good and bad ways. It can help you achieve and compete, but it can also grind you into the dirt.

- Most ambitious men attract stress but don't handle it well.

- Don't consider stress as scattered hassles and problems. Instead, step back and look at stress as a single force with competing good and bad aspects.

- The best way to manage and redirect stress is by improving your mental and physical habits and routines. No medicine, vitamin, hair color, or can of beer is going to do that for you.

- Gradually but deliberately change your habits.

- Look for long-term solutions to your bigger problems with a clearer head so you can deal with them from a position of strength.

- Support your energy level by maintaining better physical, dietary, and grooming routines.

- Enjoy your life more each day as you see the benefits of controlling stress for the many great years ahead.

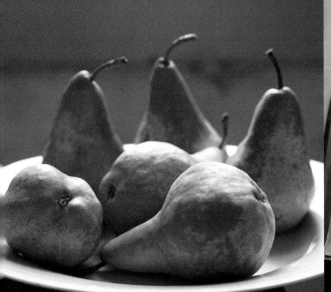

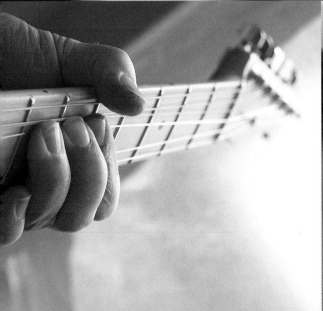

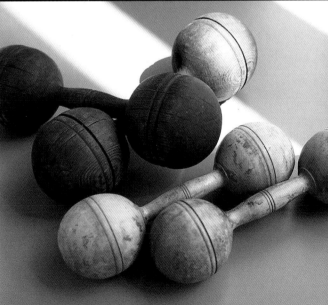

YOUR LIFE: TO TRADE-IN OR TO TUNE UP? Swapping your life for someone else's is a terrific romantic fantasy. That isn't possible, but if the game isn't going your way, there are options: You could join the pro circuit, the Peace Corps, or the merchant marines. You could change your identity, run away, and start your life over. You could take the back-to-earth approach, trying to scratch out subsistence on some remote patch of dirt. Or you could start a program of deep and expensive psychotherapy. You could even become criminally irresponsible and let the state take care of your room and board. But would your life be better?

No one's life is perfect, but if you are generally satisfied with the direction you are going, all you really need is a good tune-up. You can make those adjustments yourself. A few parts may need special attention, or even major overhaul, but when you really think about it, you probably have what you need to bring yourself up to fresh or restored glory.

Get help if you need it. If you are deeply unhappy with fundamental aspects of your life, you should seek professional counseling—particularly if you suspect depression, chemical imbalance, or serious emotional distress. Your problems are probably beyond the reach of a good massage.

What Makes Us Crazy?

There are many causes of stress, but here are six big ones:

- Lack of money. Even very wealthy men become anxious worrying about money.

- Lack of time. Few men ever feel they have enough time to spend with their family or friends, having fun, or even working.

- Too many obligations. Unless you manage time exceptionally well, it is easy to accept more responsibilities than any man has time to do well.

- A lack of control. There is a big difference between being a control freak and wanting order.

- Physical anxieties. Being overweight, suffering from common ailments, and growing less physically active and fit can drag anyone down.

- Being lonely. It's not fun. It's not healthy.

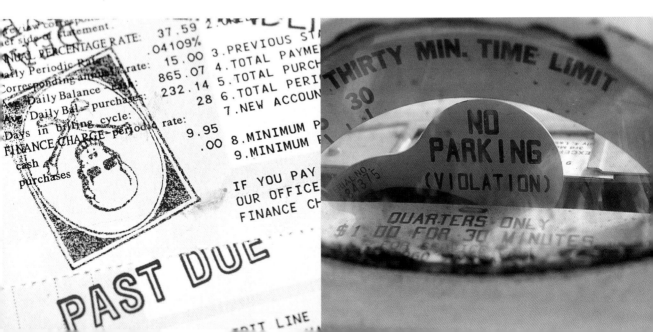

Forms Stress Takes

Stress can appear as physical annoyances that are often ineffectively treated as isolated medical problems.

Look in your medicine chest. Do you own every medication—prescribed or over-the-counter—for most common complaints? Perhaps your aches, pains, itching, insomnia, allergies, upset stomach, and cold sores result from stress, not a defective or fragile system. These complaints are easier to control and eliminate when you've identified their source, rather than as isolated and disturbing ailments. Life is simpler without unnecessary medications and products.

Common Manifestations of Stress

- Headaches
- Eye twitches
- Toothaches
- Clenching
- Biting lip, inside of mouth
- Cold sores
- Tight neck and shoulders

- Heavy sighing
- Shallow breathing
- Back pain
- Digestive distress
- Impotency
- Insomnia
- Panic attacks
- Chewing fingernails

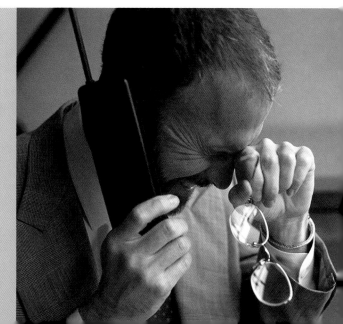

When a new symptom crops up, first consider stress as the possible cause. Start from the head and work down, and look at some of the many ways stress can get to you. Each following section starts with a description of the symptom and some easy, effective remedies, but if you find that you are frequently experiencing many of these problems, you may have some serious stress in your life, and you will need to take some steps to deal with the bigger picture. If you suspect serious illness or injury, see your medical professional.

Stress can be clever; its symptoms can migrate, and its timing can fool you. One week, you could have intense headaches. A month later no headaches, but your left shoulder is locked solid. Then insomnia pays a call. The symptoms change, but the root cause is the same—you are stressed, and you need to deal with it. Instead of getting more stressed about an illusionary medical problem, learn to identify how you exhibit stress so you can treat it directly. This is fundamental to gain control and manage stress.

Stress doesn't mirror your schedule either. Sometimes you may feel it before a big project or presentation. The next time, afterward. Some stress crops up long after it should logically appear. Consider this when you notice the next ache or twitch. Relax, nod to yourself, and know that it will be gone soon, and perhaps migrate somewhere else tomorrow. But it won't make you crazy. You are learning to redirect your stress.

Your headaches, face muscles, and toothaches

There is nothing simple about your head. Leaving aside your consciousness and psyche, your head is a sophisticated unit of moving parts, optics, electronics, chemistry, sensors, tools, processors, scanners, and input and output devices. No computer is as complicated or as fragile. Monitor your head for signs of fatigue, wear and tear, and overload. Treat it well.

As bad as hangovers can be, headaches are even worse when you don't know their cause. Their forms are not static. Following are their most common forms.

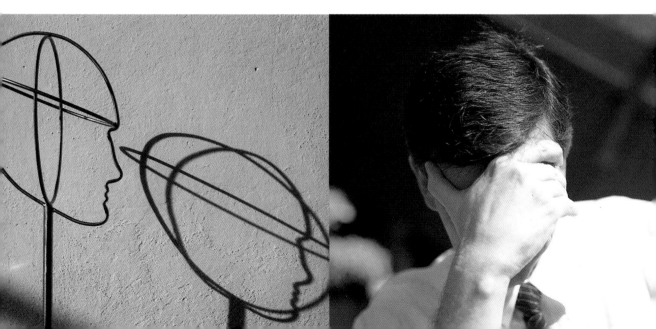

MUSCULAR OR TENSION HEADACHES are caused by injury or by stress. In fact, more than 90 percent of headaches are tension headaches. An easy way to tell if yours is one is to rub the areas that hurt. Slowly but firmly massage the sensitive parts. If you can make it feel better while you are massaging the pain, your headache is probably muscular, and probably stress-related.

To treat a muscular headache, pinpoint the areas where they occur. Unlike muscles in other parts of your body, most head muscles are finer and close to the surface. You can feel and massage most of them yourself. You will discover that your head has small muscles in unexpected places. Your temples are frequent focal points, but try rubbing the bridge of your nose, your forehead, and just above and below your eyebrows. You may be surprised at how many tiny but strong muscles it takes to keep your face working, and how tight and sore each one of them can get. They need more blood flowing through them to loosen and restore them to a more relaxed state.

Aspirin and other analgesics may help but won't be as effective if the muscles are too tight and blood flow is restricted. Slow, extended stretching, massage, and exercise can help. Working those tiny muscles with your fingertips, or even a pencil eraser, can work wonders. Check out your neck and shoulder muscles too; when they are tight, they can tighten everything up the ladder (see pages 105–106).

Mild to vigorous exercise should help a muscular headache, but if exercise makes the pain worse and you feel pulse pain—throbbing, sharp stabs that match your pulse—stop what you are doing and consider other causes.

DENTAL ACHES AND HEADACHES are deceptive. We tend to think of our teeth as solid units that hurt only when they are decayed or cracked. Instead, each tooth is individually wired to our gums, jaw, sinuses, and skull. Too much pressure on them transfers to our nerves, tightening our muscles and triggering other discomfort, often not even in our mouth. Some sinus and other nonspecific facial pain, for example, may actually be caused by clenching and grinding our teeth. If your jaw and tongue are tight, or your teeth are generally sensitive, you could be clenching.

You don't have to be awake to clench and grind. In fact, you probably cause more stress on your teeth at night than you do during the day. Stretch your jaw frequently and ask your dentist about fitting you for a mouthpiece if you notice these symptoms.

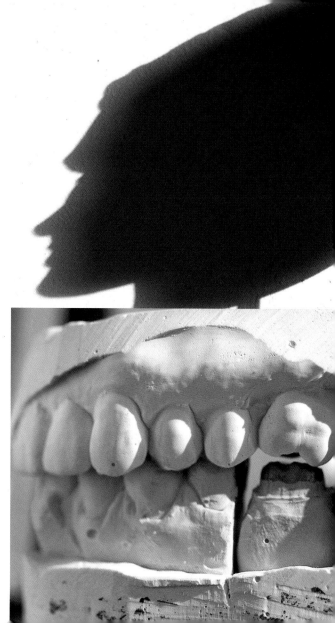

Your tongue is a powerful muscle. Though it doesn't usually feel aches, it can cause them elsewhere in your head by tightening and by putting pressure on the roof of your mouth or front teeth. It feels good to stick out your tongue occasionally, but don't do it in public.

Have you ever gone to the dentist with a specific tooth troubling you, but X-rays or an exam reveal nothing unusual? The physics of your jaw may put more pressure on that tooth that week, so it hurts more. Teeth move around; you can feel that when you floss: what's tight today is loose tomorrow. What hurts this week may not next.

One business executive noticed he always seemed to be in the dental chair with complaints of tooth pain right before important overseas trips. Eventually, it dawned on him that the pain was stress-related, and he redirected it. Now, his normal dental check-ups are all he needs.

VASCULAR HEADACHES hurt with each heartbeat. If yours is caused by a hangover, your blood vessels are constricting because you are dehydrated. Your system is trying to grab more oxygen in restricted space. Your nerves feel it, causing your head to hurt. Besides alcohol, there are other causes of pulse headaches, including high blood pressure and incorrect medications, and you should take them seriously. If you have frequent hangovers, you could be heading toward alcoholism, which is much harder to treat than a stress headache.

And if alcohol isn't to blame, you may not be drinking enough water. Beverages with caffeine and sodium—and that includes most soft drinks—do little to keep you properly hydrated.

DIET HEADACHES are caused by not eating properly, and they can have an effect similar to pulse headaches. You've heard it a million times, and it's true: you need to eat properly, and a normal-sized male body needs a minimum of 1,300 calories to maintain itself. Dehydration can also cause headaches. Make sure to drink enough fluid every day, especially in the heat.

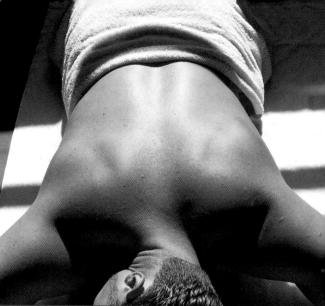

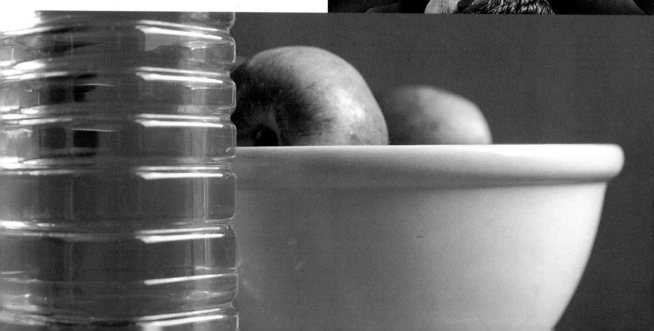

Tight muscles, shoulders, neck, back

Bad posture can cause headaches and neck, shoulder, and back pain. Chances are, you spend more time at a keyboard than your father did, and your shoulders and neck are paying a price for it. If you spend several hours at a stretch at a computer, notice if your shoulders creep up as you work. It is a wonder your shoulders don't end up in your ears! That much tension concentrated in one place will eventually lead to a painful, stiff neck. It may be triggered by something else, like getting out of bed abruptly or yanking on something suddenly, but your computer posture may have primed you for this kind of injury.

Nearly everyone has office, factory, driving, or home posture that could use improvement. Although pain is great for chiropractors, much pain can be prevented with basic good sense alone.

- Do you cradle the telephone between your neck and shoulder for long stretches?

- Is your work area set up to the right heights, angles, and distances? Tailor your workspace to your body and habits.

- Do you have to stretch to use your computer mouse?

- Do you stand and stretch at least once an hour?

- Do you slouch through your days, even when you feel good?

- Do you usually sit without both feet firmly on the floor, or with your legs crossed, for long streches?

- Has pulling your gut in as you sit, or even sitting straight in a chair, become an unusual sensation?

- Have your abs gone to hell? If so, and especially if you are overweight, your vertebrae are being torqued and will eventually cause you back pain.

All of these bad habits can eventually cause you unnecessary pain. What you need to concentrate on is better posture. You may have heard your mother tell you to stand up straight a million times when you were younger, but guess what? She was right. And not only will you look and feel better, you'll be better at all the things you enjoy—sports, sex, and even sleep.

Good posture has many benefits, all of which help eliminate or redirect stress. It makes you look and feel better and more confident instantly. Good posture keeps your circulation system flowing properly throughout your body so each part of you gets the blood it needs to stay healthy, and it helps keep your weight properly distributed so you keep the load on your muscles, vertebrae, and joints evenly balanced.

The rules of good posture are as simple today as they ever were:

- Sit up straight, stomach in, chest out, shoulders back.

- Put your feet flat on the floor when you sit.

- Keep the weight of your head balanced on your shoulders.

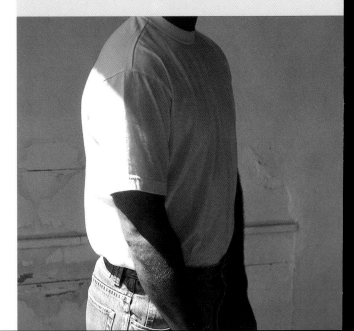

TAKE A BREATH: Take a deep breath. And another. And one or two more. Is this a new sensation too? It shouldn't be, but when we get stressed our breathing becomes shallow and quick. Excessive yawning and sighing are ways our body forces us to clear out our lungs and get a full helping of fresh air occasionally, but by then it's a little late. Several times a day, stop and take a few deep breaths. Combine that with a simple shoulder stretch to your ears when you inhale. Hold it, and then drop your shoulders all the way back when you exhale. It feels good.

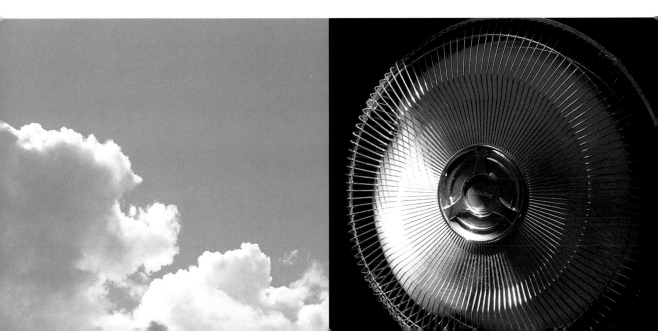

SINUS OBSESSION: As a culture, we have become sinus obsessed. The money we spend on treating the symptoms of allergies, hay fever, colds, and sinus headaches is astounding, and much of it is probably unnecessary. Instead of dosing yourself with sinus medicines, try letting your sinuses do what they are supposed to do naturally: wash and filter irritants out of your system.

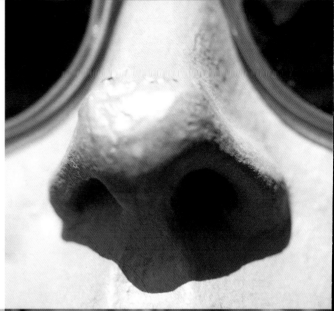

- Don't overblow your nose.

- Don't rub your eyes, as this just pushes pollen and other irritants into your mucus membranes and bloodstream.

- Don't expect your sinuses to be perfectly clear every day. By relaxing and allowing your nose to run and your eyes to water, you may discover the symptoms pass more quickly than with a regimen of allergy shots or pharmaceuticals that only masks the symptoms and may stretch out your discomfort.

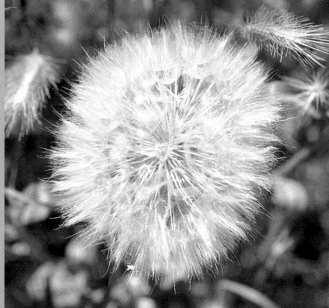

Sleep better

A few very successful men can get by on only a few hours of sleep every night. In fact, most men need lots of sleep—much more than we actually get. Recent sleep studies indicate that as a culture we are sleeping, on average, far less than we should and than our ancestors did. We have plenty of light and too many things to do, so we allow the urgency of life to keep us up well past our bedtimes.

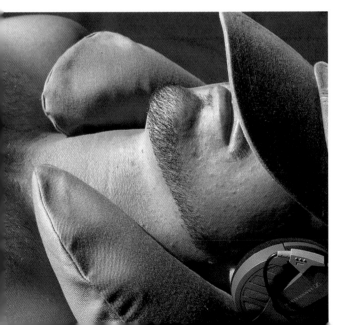

Nor do we depend on seasonal changes to set our routines. Some scientists say that we should follow the sun's rise and set to determine our daily schedules: get up with the sun, go to bed when it sets. In the winter, we would sleep for fourteen hours; in the summer, as little as seven.

That's absurd for any man who isn't a hermit, but it is a good reminder that a steady routine of six and a half hours isn't enough. Aside from obvious fatigue, drowsiness, and a lack of energy, other signs of sleep deprivation include rashes, dark under-eye circles, eyelid twitching, frequent tripping, unusual clumsiness, and becoming accident prone. Your mouth pays for your late-night fun too. If you have been biting your tongue, lip, or the inside of your mouth, chances are you need more sleep.

Tips for Establishing Better Sleep Patterns
at Home or on the Road

- Don't eat a large meal before bed, but don't go hungry either. A glass of milk sometimes helps because of the amino acids it contains.

- Soak in a long, hot bath right before bed.

- Make sure your room is as dark and quiet as you can make it. If you live somewhere noisy, you can create your own white noise with a small fan. It helps mask motor noises. Or wear foam earplugs.

- Sleep regular hours, even on the weekend. Sleeping in Sunday morning can make it harder to fall asleep Sunday night, which makes it harder to get up Monday morning, and your cycle is skewed for another week.

- If you are in a pattern of lying awake fretting about a few relatively small problems, write them down before you turn out the lights, roll over, and then focus on things that are going well. Negative thoughts trigger slight adrenaline rushes, which do nothing to relax you.

- If you can't get the problems out of your head, imagine them written down on Rolodex cards, sorted, and filed. Flip through other problem cards. Select an easier unsolved problem—everyone's got one. Exchange one for the other. It helps.

- If there is ever a time to allow yourself to feel sensual, lying in bed is one. Feel the warmth of your sleeping partner, the bedding, the dark, the calm, and the quiet. Like being in a pool of warm water, bedtime is one of the few times every square inch of your skin feels good. Remember how good your bed feels when you are waking up from a good sleep. Imagine that feeling as you try to doze off.

- To make your trip to sleep more interesting, fantasize about anything along the way. Go ahead—it's your imagination.

- Be considerate: save emotional conversations with your partner for daytime.

- Sleep on the couch when you are keeping your partner awake.

SLEEP APNEA: Extra flesh in the throat causes sleep apnea. Middle-aged, heavy men are prone to this problem, especially if they drink before bed. Heavy snorers may also suffer from this. Here's how it works: when you relax and start to fall asleep, this fatty tissue sags and cuts off your air supply, causing you to wake up frequently—sometimes many, many times a night. You may not even be aware of this happening. Not only are you not getting a good night's sleep, this can eventually lead to serious heart problems. Surgical procedures to correct this used to be dramatic, but less heroic procedures are available now.

JET LAG: The only time jet lag feels good is after a grueling flight, say from L.A. to Tokyo, arriving at your hotel room in the late afternoon, soaking in a deep tub, and crawling into a freshly made bed. Although completely wiped out, you drift off knowing that you don't have to get up for at least twelve hours. That never happens at home!

Jet lag is a serious physical reality. The following suggestions help the business traveler, but some can be applied at home.

- The best remedy is prevention. Though it may seem near impossible, try to be well rested, focused, and organized before you leave on a trip. Pretrip stress and sleep debt often intensify the sleeplessness at your destination, especially for long west-east trips.

- Don't drink alcohol before, during, or after the flight. Long flights suck moisture from your body, and alcohol speeds that process. Be careful with coffee if you have to sleep when you arrive. Drink lots of water en route, and eat lightly. Go easy on the salty nuts and pretzels. Just as they make you thirstier in a tavern, so do they when you are cruising the jet stream.

- As you settle into your seat on the plane, set your watch to the time at your destination and think of yourself in that time zone. Don't even think about what time it is back home, except when you are calling the office or your family. Some of the jet lag is a head game: presume victory.

- Most travelers find it easier to adjust when flying west: it's easier to stay awake when you are a little tired than to fall asleep a few hours earlier than your body thinks it should.

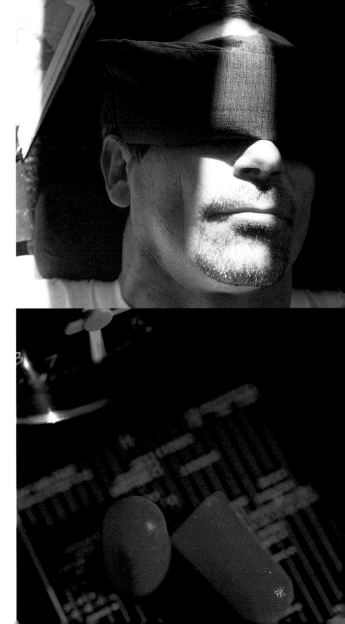

- Although you may feel okay in the days following a long trip, your body's systems take a day per time zone to get back in sync completely.

- If you can sleep on the plane, you are fortunate. It can be an efficient way to catch up on minor sleep debt. But knocking yourself out with medication for a long flight may increase the chances for insomnia at your destination.

- If you can't really sleep, a long zone-out will still help.

- Pack eyeshades, an inflatable neck pillow, and earplugs. They are effective on the plane and do double duty in a noisy or bright hotel room.

- Earplugs, though, don't cut enough of the low drone of the jet engines. You can create masking white noise by wearing music headsets over your earplugs and turning on music—any music—so low that it sounds miles away. It may seem like a stupid idea, but it works.

- You know your reading habits, but even if you have good intentions to tackle difficult reading on the plane, pack a cheesy thriller just in case. For most travelers, an exciting novel can speed a flight. Or take a stack of unread mail or magazines with you and toss them as you go. If you really need to keep an article, slice it out and toss the rest.

On arrival, here are some basic tips:

- When making a long trip, keep your postarrival activities to a minimum. Working out, taking a walk around the hotel to get your bearings and to spot a comfortable place for coffee and the newspaper the next morning, quietly settling in to the hotel, or reviewing the next day's business may not be that exciting, but you'll be in much better form the next day than if you hit a few nightspots.

- If you suffer from severe jet lag regularly, there are self-directed programs to help. They require precise control of your light levels, diet, and timing doses of melatonin before, during, and after your arrival according to the number of time zones crossed and direction traveled.

- Beware of television right before bed. Its bursts of flashing light can fool the pineal gland (the gland that releases melatonin into the body according to perceived light fields) into thinking it is daytime. Try to find some relaxing music on the radio instead, and play it quietly, so it sounds as if it is coming from a long way off.

- To reset your internal clock fast, without drugs, spend as much time as possible in full daylight without sunglasses. Studies on travelers between Australia and Los Angeles proved that two hours of exposure to sunlight was more effective than medication in speeding the transition between time zones. Recent studies have even demonstrated that skin itself may play a role in keeping your system's clock in sync.

- Resign yourself to knowing that you are going to be drowsy and out of sync for two or three days, and try to schedule your activities accordingly.

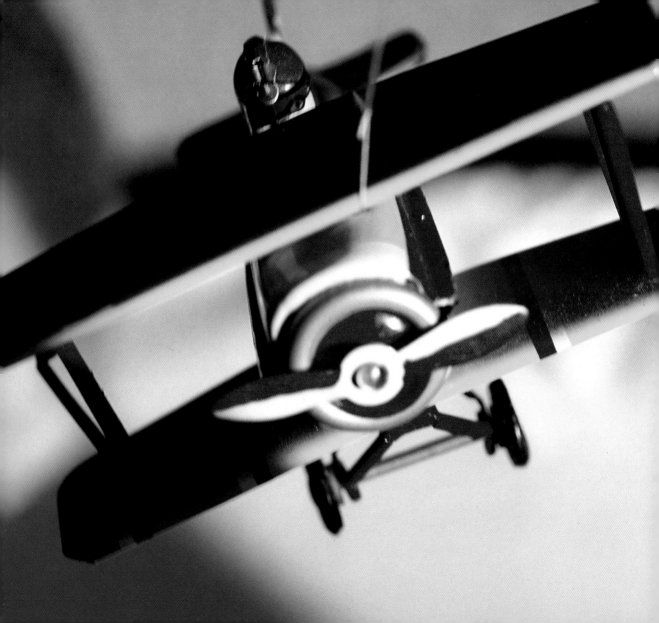

A Perfect Flight

Time in suspension. Some men use a long flight as a stretch of pure, sweet time uninterrupted by the telephone and office or family distractions. They set up their arrangements to make their trip as quiet, as comfortable, as relaxing, or as productive as they can, and then let things play themselves out. Seeing the world from cruising altitude can't help but give you more perspective on the big picture, on your career, on your relationships. Those few hours to yourself can make you feel much more in control.

You've made and confirmed all of your travel arrangements, including seat assignments, well in advance. Perhaps you've splurged on an upgrade. Maybe you aren't even exhausted. You packed well, your baggage is checked, and you have a briefcase neatly stuffed with work you feel like doing, with mail, magazines, or a book you've wanted to read. (Don't count on music—especially good, subtle jazz or classical—to ever sound as good on a plane as you want it to. Unless you have full cup earphones, the dynamic range is no match for jet engines.)

Feeling social? You could check out your seatmate, but beware—it's a lot harder to end a conversation than it is to start one. Leave the flight attendants alone; they aren't interested, and neither are you. Just enjoy spending the time with yourself.

If a movie is showing that you've been planning to see, great. If not, ignore the urge to watch—it's mostly TV and advertising that you get too much of at home.

Although aisle seats have advantages, sometimes, on clear, sunny days, just staring out the window at the patchwork below is more refreshing than anything, and worth occasionally having to step over your neighbor.

You know what you like. Allow yourself the pleasure. Why not?

Major Relaxation

Most stressed men could drive efficiency experts crazy. Citing a lack of time, many guys won't take preventive relaxation, and this is a false economy. When stress takes its toll, repair takes much longer than prevention would have, and over time you pay for it with more serious health problems. Massage, saunas, steam baths, hot baths, showers, and soaks are all effective ways to reduce stress and prevent and treat muscular aches, pains, injuries, and seizures.

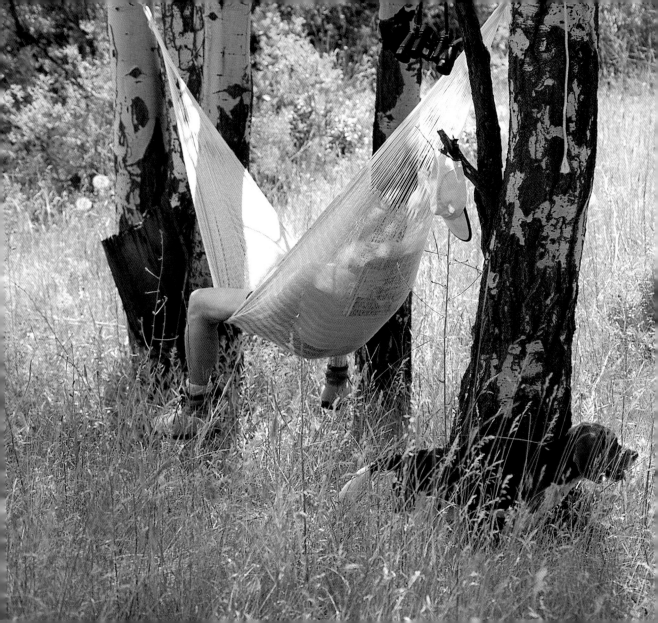

ACTIVE AND PASSIVE RELAXATION:
If you work out and get regular exercise, you already enjoy the benefits of better circulation and respiration and improved muscle tone and coordination, and you probably have a better perspective on life. Obviously, active forms of relaxation can be healthy and beneficial, but passive forms have their place too. It's fun to explore and enjoy relaxing methods to cut through stress in healthy ways.

INTERNATIONAL BATHING: Many cultures around the world know their baths. Japanese men from all professions end their long, grueling days soaking in a tub of very hot water. Traditionally, they would visit the neighborhood bathhouse, but deep home tubs are becoming the norm now. First, they sit on a stool in front of a low spigot, with a bucket, soap, a thin band of cotton towel, and a brush. And they scrub. And scrub, making sure every part of their bodies is clean,

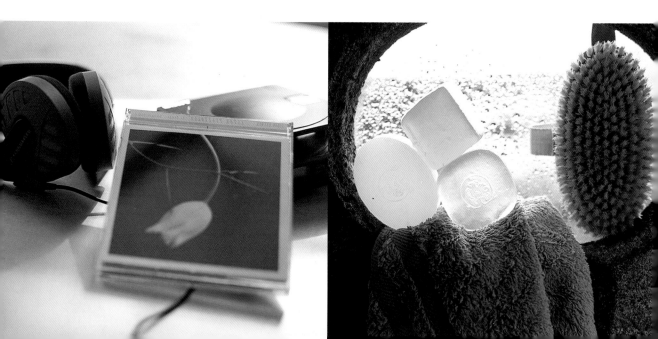

that every muscle, every hair, is properly washed and rinsed. Then, they soak. And soak. And soak. Go to a Japanese public bath, and you can sense the great release of tension as these guys let the almost scalding water heat, soften, and relax their muscles. Then they head to bed for a deep sleep. Unfortunately, the United States doesn't have an equivalent for that kind of preventive relaxation.

The Japanese take their bathing very seriously and build entire spa towns called *onsen*, built around hot springs to provide getaways for the dangerously stressed. Some have unusual features, including sand baths, in which all of you except your hands and head is buried in steaming sand—like a steam bath, but more intense under the weight and pressure of the sand. Some even feature pools with a mild electrical charge—an acquired taste.

Turkish baths are legendary, and they are still common in modern Istanbul. The first part of the routine is similar to that in Japan: scrub and rinse. But instead of a soak, the scrub is followed by lying on a large, slightly convex heated marble slab in the center of the room. The heat radiates up and through your body. Eventually, a burly guy comes along and beats you up. With sudsy water and a towel, he vigorously scrubs you down, pulling your limbs in many unlikely directions. Then, in one swift pull and squeeze, he forces blood down the length of your arm from shoulder to fingertips, for a surprising jolt to the circulation. Being kneaded like a lump of tough dough is deeply relaxing, and occasional surrender to this kind of brutal refreshment can be habit-forming— as dozens of generations of Turks have known.

In most other countries it is possible to find some suitable form of massage. Major hotels can usually recommend legitimate services and facilities.

As stress causes muscles to tense up, circulation is cut off, causing additional tension. Eventually, your muscles are so tight that nerves start to object, and your system responds by locking the muscles into bundles. Like tight knots, these are difficult to break down and soften. There are many styles of massage—most of them mellower than what the Turks mete out—but they all share a basic concept: maintain and improve circulation within your muscles to keep them pliable through movement and focused pressure that they don't get in daily activity. In the West, the most common kinds of legitimate massage include:

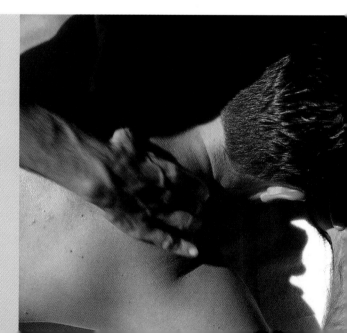

• Swedish: The traditional style, working muscles and joints by kneading pressure in the direction of the heart. This helps circulation and improves removal of metabolic waste.

• Sports: A more focused variation of Swedish massage designed as injury therapy.

• Shiatsu and Acupressure: Asian-style massage that works through applied pressure to specific "energy points" throughout the body. It is usually done fully clothed, but variations exist.

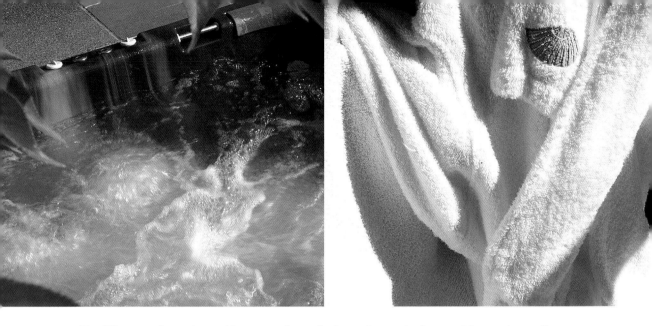

Try different styles and practitioners until you find one that works for you. Massage is usually performed in half-hour blocks; indulge for an hour if you can tell that the tension is getting out of control. If you like more forceful pressure, let the masseuse know. If there are specific areas that are bothering you, identify them.

If you are squeamish about trying a massage for the first time, try one of the chain stores that give short massages to fully clothed customers.

PROFESSIONAL SPAS AND FACILITIES: If you are lucky enough to have access to a gym or facility that offers soaking and massage, great. But many massage therapists practice in office suites without showers or baths. That's fine, and much better than no massage at all. But more men are enjoying the benefits of full-on, Swiss-style spas for major rest and recuperation. These don't come cheap, but it can be well worth it if you are suffering from major stress.

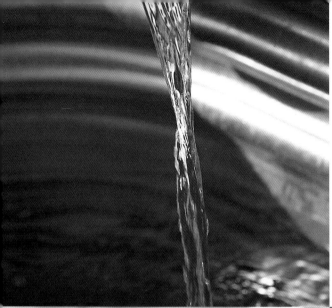

HOME SPA IDEAS: Hot tubs have been popular in American homes since the 1960s, and some of them would put anything in the Playboy mansion to shame. If you can afford it, fine, but lots of guys can experience similar benefits in a plain old bathtub. Here are some suggestions:

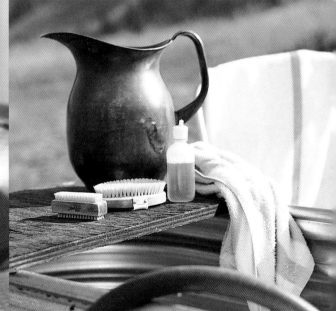

- Without hot water, you don't have much of a spa. The other essential ingredients are a little time to let the water do the trick and some peace and quiet.

- Salts, soaps, and scrub brushes are terrific. In Europe, green liquid kelp soap is as common as Ivory, and it has a great soothing, slightly medicinal smell. The stuff isn't hard to find in health food stores or shops that sell natural soaps and oils.

- Can't find someone to give you a massage or to scrub your back? A long-handled brush will have to suffice. Remember that you are trying to invigorate your skin and circulation, not peel it away like a layer of old paint, so go easy.

- Massage oils can be especially soothing.

- If you float long enough to let the water cool, drain some and refill the tub. A typical soak for Japanese in a bathhouse is at least a half hour, so be sure you are giving yourself enough time for the soothing forces of the hot water to do their work.

- Bring a magazine or book, daydream, or doze if you can do it without slipping below the water line.

- Block out visual distractions with eyeshades and really listen to a long jazz or classical album.

- Be careful as you get out, and hold on to the side of the tub in case you get a little light-headed, which is common. Shower to rinse off the soap and residue, then towel off and wrap yourself in a bathrobe.

- The main thing is to enjoy yourself and reclaim some control over your body. You will sleep more soundly, and wake up better prepared to reenter the battle for another round.

- Finally, promise yourself that you'll cut yourself enough slack to do this—or something just as relaxing—every few weeks.

Turning Bad Habits into Good Patterns

Habits are individual acts; patterns are strings of habitual behavior. From the day we are born, they form the basis of our actions, providing comfort, routine, safety, and efficiency. But not all habits are good: excessive drinking or smoking; poor diet; abusive behavior to ourselves, loved ones, or strangers; dishonesty and disrespect. Most men understand the difference between good habits and bad but find that the randomness and chaos of the day—demands at home and at work—can create an atmosphere of urgency that encourages an erosion of good habits. Over time, the discipline of maintaining good habits is compromised until they are reduced to good intentions—eventually sliding into bad habits and negative patterns. We lose self-control and slip into a coping mode. It may not kill us quickly, but it isn't healthy.

Bad habits can change for the better, especially taken on one at a time. Improved habits can be strung together into successful patterns. Despite the old saw that you can't teach old dogs new tricks, many men find that it is actually easier to change some habits and patterns as one gets older. In adolescence and young adulthood, peer pressure compels us to try unhealthy stunts—like playing chicken, binge drinking, all-nighters, and bungee jumping. The older you get, the less attractive this risky behavior seems. Most smokers, for example, start in their early teens. When you outgrow the urge to "be cool," you can prevent many bad habits from becoming ingrained. Maturity has some advantages; this is one of them.

IMPROVING BAD HABITS: Small changes add up. Here are some basic techniques to help deal with annoying daily habits. As each habit—no matter how minor—is improved, it creates and then reinforces a pattern of success and reward.

- Take small steps to improve the organization in your life. We all know how annoying it is to regularly lose items we use every day—misplaced keys, for example, or airline tickets, an appointment book, sunglasses, or an umbrella. Assign a single spot to each item—the same pocket for keys, a compartment of your briefcase for airline tickets, a spot on your desk for your appointment book or sunglasses, a place by the front door for your umbrella—and return it to that place whenever you put it down. If you are on a business trip, enforce the same patterns. Your hotel key goes into the same pocket; your umbrella in a place close to the front door in your hotel room. It's simple, but it works.

- Carry that kind of organization into other parts of your life—your desk or tool bench, gym bag, tackle box, glove compartment, bills-to-pay folder, parking place, and where you put your parking stub or dry cleaner receipt.

- Write down computer default settings, passwords, and customized instructions and keep them in the same place near your computer so you don't waste time and energy looking for them. (Perhaps, as it does with jokes, our mind stores this data in a portion of our brain that is frequently purged!)

- Create a yearly calendar—preferably on a single page—to keep track of important dates and to develop a long-range vision of your immediate future. Besides anniversaries and birthdays, include things like driver's license and passport renewal dates, and insurance and property tax due dates.

- If you are consistently shy about asking for driving directions somewhere, resolve to get over that—or buy a road map and use it.

You know how easy it could be to improve these habits and so many more. So why wait? Resolve to reduce fundamental stress and frustration and use the following tips:

- Organize your closets, eliminating clothes or items you haven't worn or used in two years.

- Organize your desk.

- Devise a simple filing system that works for you.

- Shop smarter by making lists and keeping receipts.

- Plan your days, weeks, months, and vacations in advance.

- Schedule routine maintenance for your car.

- Keep track of telephone numbers and addresses in a convenient place.

- Always read (or at least skim) operating or assembly instructions for an appliance, so when you run into a problem, you know where the answer might be.

- Call the airport to see if the flight you are meeting is on time.

- Confirm important professional and personal appointments.

- Remember important dates and anniversaries.

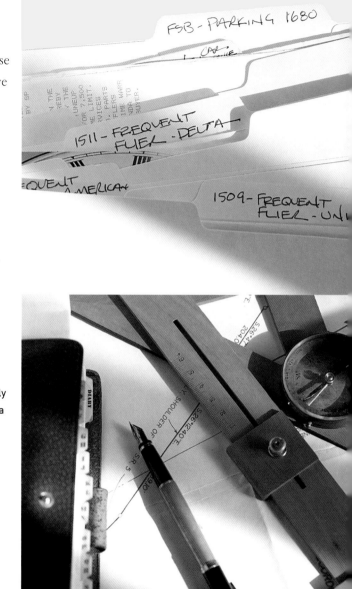

IS YOUR LIFE READY FOR A DATABASE? The best organization system is one that you will use consistently, year in and year out. One busy man discovered that by using a simple database program on his computer, he could keep all of the paper in his life organized, off his desk, yet easy to locate when he needs it. Once you understand the system's underlying logic, you can tailor it to suit your own requirements. Here's his plan.

- First, buy a box or two of file folders.

- Clean out your old files and toss any that you know you will never need again.

- With the remainder, group them in any way that makes sense for your life—Auto, Home, Personal Documents, Taxes, Travel, Bills to Pay, Bills Paid, etc.

- File your records into the folders and number them according to the categories you created. You don't have to be very careful about this numbering system—that's where the beauty of the database comes in.

- Create a file in the database program and set up a numbering system that corresponds with your file folders. In descriptive fields, describe the contents of your folders using simple key words such as Federal Tax Records—1999–2002; Dental Insurance Policy; Family Birth Certificates; or Retirement Program.

- Describe the contents with a few tag words. They need to be descriptive enough to help you locate them in the future. For example, let's take travel award program literature that you may need to retrieve. Instead of stuffing it in a file and marking it "Travel Awards," assign it a number and describe it in your database with keywords like Travel, Awards, Frequent Flier, or any other you want.

- Put the folders in numerical order in your file cabinet. When you need to find that file, you can search the database using the keywords to locate the correct file's assigned number. No matter where it is or how the number is assigned, you can quickly locate that file. (Of course, you can number the file folders into some logical grouping if that suits your temperament, but that's optional.)

- Add new folders or use existing ones each time you receive a new document to file.

ESTABLISHING SUCCESSFUL ROUTINES:
Look for routine structures that work for you and maintain them so that you don't have to stop and retrace your steps. You don't have to flip into a frustration mode several times a day; instead, create a pattern of successful patterns. That's what you need to start redirecting bad stress.

Have you ever noticed that you get a slight mental hit when you find something you often lose just where you deliberately put it? That buzz is good. The more aspects of your life you can apply this simple principle to, the less trivial frustration you will experience.

Gradually, you can move to more difficult physical habits. Like regular exercise, for example. Do you ever regret working out? Probably not. In fact, if most men could get a hint of the buzz they feel after a workout beforehand, they would find physical exercise as pleasurable as eating or drinking. Athletes and gym rats do anticipate this charge, which hooks them into their routines. Follow their lead.

So how do you develop a pattern of regular exercise? Like the ad says, "Just do it." One especially disciplined and successful middle-aged woman in Seattle gets up nearly every morning at 5:30 A.M. so she can row on the lake by 6:00. She has an attitude most people should emulate. Her simple advice: "I don't think about it, because if I did, I'd stay in bed. I head out the door. Before I know it, I am enjoying my favorite part of the day. As soon as I wake up, I consider the decision already made." She's tough, and she's right.

You don't have to be an athlete to get a similar charge. If you don't have an established exercise or gym routine, start basic, even if it's just a brisk, regular walk around the neighborhood before breakfast or after dinner. As with your car battery, you can generate more energy moving than parked. Expend no energy thinking of excuses. Instead, just do it, and start building from there.

BREAKING CRAVINGS: Habits are simple, while cravings are more difficult, and addictions are very serious business. Recent research has revealed that our bodies actually rewire themselves to accommodate addiction to drugs. Nerve structures physically change. In part, this explains why serious addictions are so difficult to break. But they can be broken, especially with good professional help and support. Earlier is always better. In contrast to addiction, getting the better of cravings is simple.

- Recognize the craving you want to break.

- Decide how serious you are.

- Proceed only on ones that you really want to change. Frequent backsliding sets up other negative patterns that do no good. You need to put 100 percent into this.

- Design a strategy that is likely to work, and set up rewards for yourself when you resist the craving. For example, if you are trying to quit smoking, put yourself into nonsmoking social situations that discourage you from even considering lighting up.

- Know the times of day that the cravings are strongest and plan your schedule to subdue them. Movies are excellent distractions.

- Maintain that behavior so it becomes your normal routine.

- Enjoy the results.

Remember that the first time you deny a craving is the hardest; the second time is difficult; it gets easier the third time; and so on. Those who have successfully quit smoking, for example, are surprised that, after the first day, they actually survived. On the second, their world is not ending. They are not violently ill. They may still crave nicotine; they may be light-headed or edgy; but when they stop and do a quick check, it is not so bad, especially with well-planned distractions and a little support from friends and family.

Positive reinforcement works in a similar manner. Have you ever gone to the gym consistently and then stopped? The longer you stay away, the harder it seems to go back; your excuses and rationalizations grow more elaborate. When you do go back, once you start your old routine, it seems easy. You feel a little foolish, having stayed away so long.

START HAPPY, GET BETTER: So much of improving our lives boils down to maintaining healthy habits. All educators know how much more effective positive reinforcement is than guilt and punishment. As an adult, you are responsible for your own habits, so perhaps you should consider establishing your own rewards to improve your own behavior.

To work well, rewards must provide adequate gratification. When you were a grade school student, a gold star on a bulletin board chart may have worked magic, but as an adult, you may not be so easily reinforced. Does money work for you? Perhaps a night out? Football tickets? A few shares of stock? Here are a few ideas:

- If, for example, you want to stop eating a bowl of ice cream after every dinner, what incentive will get you to follow through? A new pair of running shoes? Great. Promise yourself that you will buy a great new pair after you have gone for a full month without eating ice cream.

- How many shares of stock is a month of beers good for?

- An hour-long massage is an excellent reward for going to the gym every night for two weeks.

- Get the car professionally detailed for cleaning out your garage, attic, basement, or office.

- Take a night class as your reward for getting a good performance evaluation.

- Buy yourself a hardcover edition of a book you've wanted to read for keeping the TV turned off after work for a week.

- Take a weekday afternoon off to take a long bike ride for landing an important new client for your company.

- Plan a hike or a weekend away with a friend or two for losing ten pounds.

Get the picture? The pattern is simple: reward good behavior with more positive perks. Don't reward good behavior with bad substitutes. Some stupid but popular rewards include cigars, drinking binges, drugs, nights with hookers, or weekends at casinos. These are not usually the wisest choices when you are trying to break bad habits.

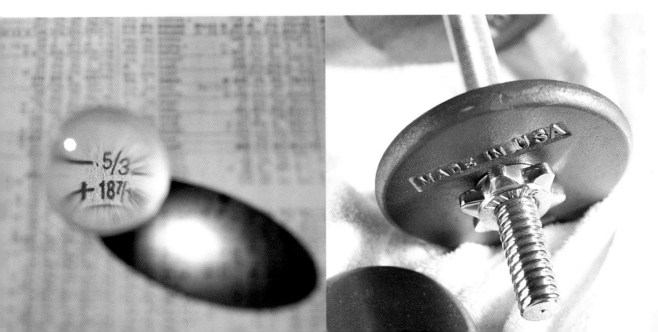

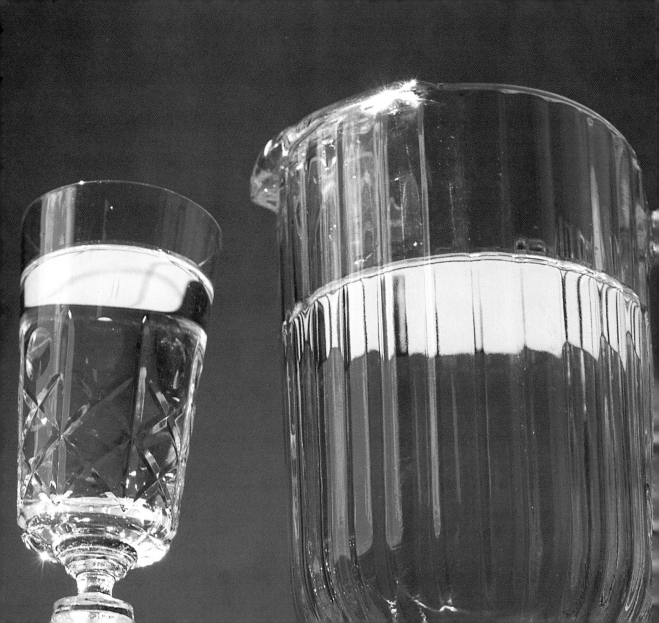

THE WATER CURE: Most addiction counselors will tell you that cravings are easier to break when you change other reinforcing habits at the same time. Smokers, for instance, associate drinking soft drinks, coffee, and liquor with smoking. As you quit smoking, quit drinking those beverages too, at least until the association is completely broken. Instead, drink a glass of water every time you want a cigarette—every time—for two to three weeks. Your bad patterns will start to break down, and your system will get a good flushing—which it probably needed.

The water cure can work for other cravings, too. Just substitute a simple glass of water for food and alcohol cravings. Instead of a cocktail or beer, drink water—plenty of it. It sounds too simple to work, but it does. Try it yourself for a few weeks. You will find yourself more in control.

A word on timing: If you can, start to work on your cravings at least a week or so before vacation instead of upon arrival. Your home pattern can be reinforced by a vacation pattern, which makes maintaining the routine after your return home that much easier.

Cravings aren't all physical. Sometimes coworkers and friends can spell trouble when you are trying to change behavior. Be disciplined and tough, and stick to your resolve. But don't make a spectacle out of yourself. You don't want to be such a jerk about your newfound virtue that those around you make it their goal to see you backslide!

HABIT EQUITY: For many men, it helps to think of building equity with good habits. Every day you pass up the superburger with 1,500 calories and 30 grams of fat is a day of credit. Every workout is a direct deposit. Every day you put in thirty minutes of aerobic exercise makes you that much stronger, that much tougher. Every day you don't drink too much, smoke, or do drugs is a day your body has to recover from previous abuse; it's a day your kidneys and liver can function normally; it's a day you can enjoy feeling a little more alert—a little more alive.

Basic, Realistic Time Management

- Inventory your time. Make a list of all the activities that claim your time in a typical day, week, and month. It's scary. If you are going to have any time to yourself, even a few hours a month to help you burn off some stress, you need to be accurate—and tough.

- Kill the tube. Television, good or bad, is a time drain. The easiest way for most of us to gain a few hours in the day is to cut down or eliminate television—or its cousin, the Internet. So much of what is broadcast is redundant that you'll hear what you missed soon enough anyway.

- Consider the traffic. Traffic everywhere, it seems, is getting worse, so it takes longer to run errands, get to work, pick up the kids, and go to a show. By making lists, planning, and applying some imagination, you may be able to pick up a few hours a week by reconsidering the times and sequences you run through your day.

- Set priorities. Eliminate parts of your daily routine that you don't enjoy anymore. Be ruthless. Look at all the ways you spend time; examine your motivations and benefits. Routine compels us to do things mindlessly.

- Look for alternatives. Do you really need to drive every morning? Could you take a train or bus and get some reading or a little planning done on the way to work? Or, instead of listening to talk-show banter on the drive into work, could you better plan your day with the aid of a little voice recorder so that by the time you arrived, most of your big decisions were already made? If you are clever, you might even be able to leave work at a reasonable time.

- Make lists. A trip to the hardware store that should take a half hour can take more than twice that if you have to return to get something you forgot.

- Exercise with your partner and the kids. You can design activities to include the family. If the kids are too young to jog with you, have them ride a bike or rollerblade. With patience, practicing any outdoor game with the kids can be a good workout. Home after dark? Go to the pool, to a lighted play field, skating, or to the gym.

- Eat lunch alone. Having lunch with friends is fine, but it always takes longer and it takes away from time with yourself. Even a half hour not talking to someone or dealing with stuff at work can be a relief.

- Plan practical vacations. If you have a week-long vacation, and it will take almost four stress-filled days getting to and from your destination, does it make sense to go at all? Instead, reconsider a suitable alternative only four or five hours away. Or accumulate vacation time so you can take a two-week vacation somewhere more exotic.

- Reconsider the annual pilgrimage. Do you have to be with the family during the holidays? Not only is it more difficult and more expensive to travel during peak seasons, it often leads to an inferior visit. Consider other times of the year to pay your dues, and it might be a better visit for everyone.

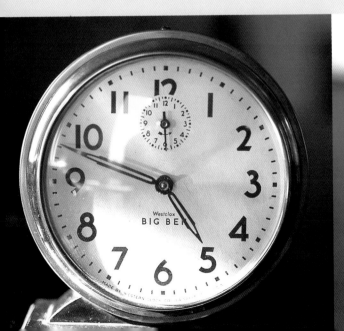

GENERAL ANXIETY: As any happy hundred-year-old will tell you, the secret to health, life, and humor is the ability to keep everything in perspective. Apply this good advice to your own life, in your own way. How will you see your job, money, relationships, and family, if you live to be a hundred?

It's not hard to see things in perspective when you take the time and think clearly. Most modern anxiety is short-term: now, today, this week. And most of the best solutions are long-term: next month, next year, in the next decade. You can make better immediate decisions when they are based on long-term goals. That's one of the many lessons maturity teaches us. But what about surviving the here and now? Here are a few pointers:

- Anxiety can be helpful. If you run a business that is having trouble, this will make you anxious. Although it doesn't feel good, this anxiety shows that you are thinking about the problem, and aren't ignoring something that needs your attention. Through this anxiety, you are more likely to come up with a solution to save the business than someone who just doesn't care.

- The secret of dread. How many times have you resisted going to a family reunion or a dental appointment, or making a difficult telephone call? And then it wasn't so bad? Our minds do help us anticipate—and even get over—distress before we actually experience it. Psychologists say that our mind works on all kinds of problems consciously and unconsciously; we may even work things out in our dreams.

- Don't take the bait. Difficult people are a given. Who makes you crazy? It may be your in-laws, your boss, an arrogant client, a lazy colleague, an old girlfriend, your brother, or even the neighbor's kid. They incite instant anger in you, and cause you to say things or behave in a way you regret. Maybe they aren't even trying to set you off—but regardless, you are in a better position when you don't take their bait.

- Pick your battles. You can control much in your life, but some things are pointless. Your sister-in-law is never going to get a new personality, so surrender. Instead of fuming, think of graceful ways to spend less time with her. Your mother may never stop treating you like a ten-year-old. So put up with it with good humor, and find ways to deflect the conversations you dislike.

- Look for resilient and successful role models. Important people in your life, either public person-alities or men and women close to you, all have jobs to do and roles to play. But they can be important role models. Resilient public figures, either contemporary or historical, are yours to learn from.

- Take charge when you can and should. Don't when you shouldn't. Throughout history there are examples of men who have assumed positions they shouldn't have. We may be attracted to new responsibility and promotion, but it does our anxiety load, and family, no good to take on jobs that others should have.

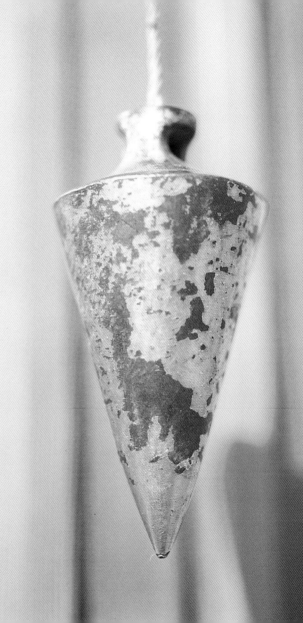

GETTING A (SOCIAL) LIFE: Loneliness is a way of life for too many single men, and the irony is that there are millions of lonely guys who want and need friendship, companionship, or romance but are clueless about how to find them.

Studies have shown that most women are much better at creating and maintaining close friendships than men are. And yet other studies have shown that most men miss friendship with other men, and they miss it a lot. Perhaps it's because friendship requires time and effort of two individuals simultaneously. Shyness certainly plays a part, too. The best way to cure shyness is to participate in group situations and activities.

Friendship at first sight is as rare as love at first sight. Repeated contact with someone is the best way to get to know that person and to let the friendship develop naturally. Friendships developed at the gym will probably last longer than those started on an airline flight or in a hotel bar. Put yourself into social situations that repeat, so you are more likely to see the same people many times, not just once. Regardless of whether you are interested in friendship, companionship, or romance, here are some places to improve your chances of meeting new people:

- Evening classes or other group instruction
- Sports teams or clubs, reading groups, civic and volunteer organizations
- Cultural groups like museums, theater, and musical clubs
- Religious services attended regularly
- Hobbyist groups
- Travel tours and outings

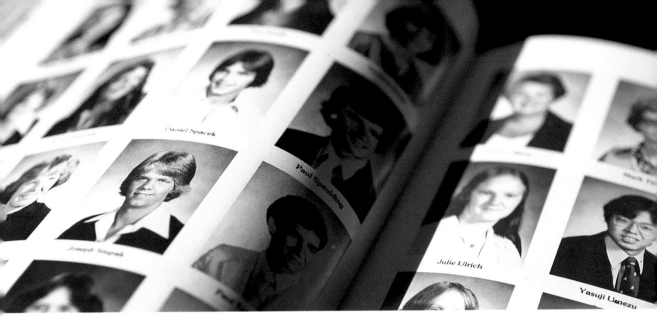

IF HIGH SCHOOL WAS THE BEST TIME OF YOUR LIFE, YOU NEED HELP!
Some friendships and other relationships are more trouble than they are worth, and if you find yourself in a endless cycle of deadhead weekends with the same stale group of buddies, hanging out at the same spots you haunted in high school, move on quick. The best friendships are those that challenge you to learn new things and develop different perspectives, and encourage you to enhance and improve your life. Those are the relationships to groom.

FAMILY FRIENDS: Some guys find themselves trapped in family or professional obligations that fill every moment of free time. For some, their best friends exist within the family. But if you are part black sheep, branch out, move away, break out of the mold that's been built around you.

BASIC ETIQUETTE: If your parents didn't do a good job of teaching you basic manners—and there is plenty of evidence that many didn't—they aren't that difficult to learn. But rather than list rules of what you should and should not do, learning the logic of etiquette will help you develop a common sense that will serve you in good stead.

Manners lubricate social transactions. We all understand the purpose of traffic and criminal laws: they prevent damage and help society run more smoothly. Manners have a similar, if more subtle, effect.

The important things to remember are that etiquette presumes a respect for others and their privacy, a base level of dignity for yourself, and simple grace as opposed to blunt efficiency. Good manners allow you to socialize comfortably in many social settings, and to enjoy yourself and your company with minimal anxiety. You can pick up good manners in any culture (including your own) by reading about them, and by observing those who use them.

Bad manners indicate an insensitivity to others. A good, simple way to improve your own is to try to observe your behavior as though you were watching yourself. Say you are waiting for an elevator in a lobby, and the doors open to reveal several passengers ready to exit. You could charge in before they have walked out, or you could stand to the side until the elevator is empty and then enter. If you were observing from a safe distance, there is no question which would be the most courteous—and most efficient. But somehow, when we are blind to the way we act, we automatically opt for the least courteous and most aggressive and disruptive behavior. The smoothest stars, though, always know how to present themselves with grace and subtle style. Their keen sensitivity to others around them allows them to look suave and assured.

Basic dinner party manners should be second nature to any guy old enough to buy a drink:

- Show up on time.

- Bring something nice for your dinner party host or hostess. It doesn't have to be expensive—a decent bottle of wine, a small bunch of flowers (probably not red roses unless you intend to signal passionate romantic interest), a box of good candy, or a book you know would be appreciated.

- Don't talk too much. Be an attentive listener, but do engage in conversation; you are more than a piece of furniture.

- Remember basic table manners. Put your napkin in your lap as soon as you sit down at the table. Eat slowly and never talk with food in your mouth.

- Leave on time; don't overstay your welcome.

- Send a thank-you card or message within a week.

Stress Control Review

Early in this chapter we listed six things that make us crazy. Let's review those and see if we can't look at each one with a healthier perspective.

- Lack of money. You aren't making enough, you are spending too much, you aren't tracking the money you do spend carefully enough, or all of the above. There are plenty of opportunities to improve your financial health, if you make a habit of following good, solid financial advice.

- Lack of time. Unless you discover a way to stretch time itself, you will have to manage what you have more thoughtfully and efficiently. Set new priorities and review them every few months to make sure you are spending the time you have in the way that makes the most sense for you. Perhaps you cut some tedious social or professional obligations to devote more time to your family or close friends.

- Too many obligations. If you are the type who says yes to every request for a favor, step back and reconsider each one carefully. Obligations take time, but they also take energy that might be better spent in other, more productive ways.

- A lack of control. Few men thrive in chaos, so work to sustain your natural level of order. Try to anticipate likely outcomes so major events—traumas like a family illness—aren't overwhelming or devastating. Plan for the inevitable.

- Physical anxieties. Some psychologists think we wear our anxieties by being overweight, out of shape, or in poor health. Anatomy may be destiny, but so is good health, and that's something you have some control over.

- Being lonely. Unless you are an incurable loner, get a social life you can enjoy.

Sex: The Good, the Bad, and the Ugly

Properly handled, dynamite is powerful and useful, but its potential for destruction always lurks. So it is with sex. Procreation aside, most men find that sexual pleasure and release are biological necessities. No other activity can provide the same physical benefits. The emotional gratification sex can provide is incomparable as well. Sex helps define you as an individual; it is an integral part of your personality, as strongly linked to you as your intellect or your body. Though sex is a highly individual and complex component of every man, there are some common fundamentals among men that relate to sex.

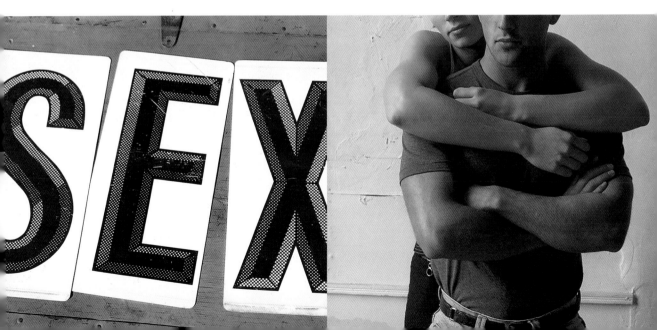

The ugly

It doesn't take much to pick up a nasty sexual disease. The physical damage caused by sexually transmitted diseases (STDs) is a profound reality. On a global scale, and on a personal one, the impact is devastating. Although a little more difficult to prevent than pregnancy, assuming a little discretion, prevention and responsibility can go a long way toward helping you and your partner live a longer, healthier life. HIV/AIDS has claimed the focus of the media in the past decade, and many sexually active men and women assume that if they can avoid that big one, they are home free. Unfortunately, it's not that simple. For starters, consider that it is over one hundred times easier to catch Hepatitis B, a potentially lethal disease. A more deadly variant, Hepatitis C, is also spreading rapidly. Other maladies multiply the risk even more dramatically. A quick flip through the sexually-transmitted diseases section of the appendix (page 157) should convince you to be very careful if you are sexually active.

PREVENTION: For both pregnancy and the spread of disease, your chances of prevention are excellent if you use a latex condom properly—every time. For now, this is the only reliable option for men who want to assume responsibility and control—as all men should (see appendix, pages 156–57). Most condoms are packaged with instructions, but the following bear repeating:

- Use only latex condoms from fresh packages that have not been damaged or exposed to chemicals, sunlight, or temperature extremes.

- Do not use oil-based lubricants (like Vaseline); they can dissolve rubber. Sterile, water-based jellies and lubricants are commonly available in pharmacies. Some brands contain spermicide to add another layer of protection.

- Wear your condom as soon as there is a possibility of exchange of any fluids; i.e. from the start of lovemaking.

- Use each one once and once only.

- Don't linger. Dispose of the condom and its contents immediately after making love.

Enhancing sexual energy

Sexual energy ebbs and flows throughout men's lifetimes. Though it may seem hard to believe when you are 18, you may not always be ready for sex anywhere and at any time. Uninspiring sexual encounters, stress, and hormonal changes can all play a part in reduced sexual drive. However, this is no cause for despair; you can and should enjoy sex well into your old age.

CHANGE YOUR ROUTINE: Even good sex between loving partners can use a boost some-times. If you find that you or your partner is not finding lovemaking satisfying enough, try experimenting a little.

- Vary the timing. If you only have sex on weekends or at night, try it during the week, in the morning, or meet for a lunch time tryst.

- Concentrate on foreplay and draw it out as long as you can. Exchange massages. Focus on less-traditional body parts; experiment with other erogenous zones like the ears, neck, navel, inner thighs, fingers, or toes.

- Shower or bathe together.

- Watch an erotic video together.

- Integrate props and toys into lovemaking.

- Try new positions.

- Exchange and act out fantasies.

Sometimes just discussing alternatives to the usual routine is enough to add spice to a lagging sex life. But remember, routine isn't necessarily a bad thing; sex between longtime partners can get better and better as you get to know your partner's likes and dislikes. Trust also enables people to experiment with things they might not have wanted to try with someone new.

STRESS: If you notice a big drop in sexual drive, it could be caused by stress. Your head is your largest and most important sex organ, and your emotions, fantasies, and personal entanglements reside there. If you sense problems, or peculiar or unusual urges that disturb you, go to a counselor. That's what they are there for. If instead, other non-sexual stresses are at work here, you may be creating an unhealthy pattern of sexual inactivity. Your sex organs, tubes, nerves, blood vessels, and muscles that make them do all the thing they do, need to be primed and active to stay healthy. As with any other part of your body, use it or lose it.

HORMONAL CHANGES: Hormonal urges that cause you to think of little else but sex during your younger years ease up somewhat as you mature. This is both a pity and a blessing, but these shifts are not usually dramatic and should not cause major physical or emotional trauma or change. If the realities of aging are the cause of your reduced performance, remember that over half of men over 40 have this problem, and if this is causing you and your partner more serious problems in your relationship, there are medical options, including Viagra and other popular medications. Designed to facilitate erections, they have captured the imagination of millions of men—perhaps to an absurd degree. (As one woman said recently, "If there is one thing the world does not need, it's more erections!") Although their reputation for success is impressive, less well-known are the side effects of these drugs, including headaches, sinus and nasal congestion, and blurred vision. Perhaps the bigger issue is that if one of these drugs works for you, are you going to need to take a pill every time you want to make love? In a culture that has grown too dependent on pharmaceuticals, do you really need a pill to help maintain fundamental human relationships? A simpler way to enhance the sex, and to help prevent urinary incontinence later in life, is to do Kegel exercises regularly. These isometric exercises strengthen the muscles in your urinary and sexual tracts and lead to greater control during sex. Strengthening these muscles will help you to maintain an erection longer—a benefit that comes with age as well—and give greater pleasure to your partner. These exercises can be done anywhere, any time. Here is how to do them:

- Locate the muscles you use to stop urine in mid-stream. These are the muscles around your urethra and anus.

- Practice squeezing them. Your stomach and buttock muscles should not move.

- Hold for three seconds. Relax for three seconds. Repeat 10–15 times per session, three times a day.

Remember that sex should be fun—enjoy yourself!

Medical Appendix

Prevention Recommendations for Adult Males

These recommendations are for the general population. Adaptations should be made based on personal risk and personal and family medical histories.

SCREENING TESTS	FREQUENCY AT VARIOUS AGES			
	18-39 yrs.	40-49 yrs.	50-65 yrs.	over 65 yrs.
General Health Review*	every 5 years	every 5 years	every 5 years	every 2 years
Hypertension	every 2 years (more often if elevated)	every 2 years (more often if elevated)	every 2 years (more often if elevated)	every 2 years (more often if elevated)
Vision	every 5 years	every 4 years	every 4 years	every 2 years
Cholesterol	—	every 5 years (more often if elevated)	every 5 years (more often if elevated)	every 5 years (more often if elevated)
Immunizations**	discuss with physician	discuss with physician	discuss with physician	discuss with physician
General Cancer Checkup	every 3 years	every year	every year	every year
Colon/Rectal Cancer	—	—	• yearly blood test and sigmoidoscopy; • periodic stool testing; • flexible sigmoi-doscopy every 3-5 years; • colonoscopy and digital rectal every 10 years	• yearly blood test and sigmoidoscopy; • periodic stool testing; • flexible sigmoi-doscopy every 3-5 years; • colonoscopy and digital rectal every 10 years
Prostate Cancer	—	—	discuss with physician	discuss with physician
Skin Cancer	every 3 years, over age 20	every year	every year	every year
Testicular Cancer	monthly self-examination (note: men ages 20-40 are at the greatest risk)	monthly self-examination	monthly self-examination	monthly self-examination
Hearing	—	—	—	once

*General Health Review

A General Health Review normally includes:

- A review of overall health and lifestyle habits
- Physical exam (including eye, ear, nose, throat, skin, heart, lungs, thyroid, and overall examination of the body)
- Screening tests (labwork, blood tests) as needed or recommended
- Immunizations as needed or recommended
- Discussion and counseling on disease and accident prevention, health promotion, health education, and healthy lifestyle habits

**Immunization Recommendations

(discuss with physician)

- Tetanus-diphtheria: every ten years
- Pneumococcal vaccine: for those at high risk of complications and infections, or for those over 65 (once in a lifetime)
- Influenza vaccine: for those at high risk of infection (every year for those over 65)
- Hepatitis: for those at high risk of infection

Although health reviews, screening tests, and immunizations are important in preventive care, the most effective form of preventive medicine may be changing lifestyle and personal health behaviors.

Men under the age of 40 are more likely to die from accidents, gunshot wounds, or injury than disease. Driving while intoxicated and failure to use seat belts are major contributors to motor vehicle injuries.

For men over the age of 40, lifestyle-related diseases remain the main causes of death. Physical inactivity, smoking, and dietary factors contribute to heart disease, cancer, diabetes and other common diseases. In the U.S. each year 455,00 men die of heart disease, 100,000 die of lung cancer and 35,000 die of prostate cancer. Men are far more likely to commit suicide, or to become addicted to drugs and alcohol.

According to the U.S. Preventive Services Task Force, "approximately half of all deaths occurring in the U.S. in 1990 may be attributed to external factors such as tobacco, alcohol, and illicit drug use, diet and activity patterns, motor vehicles, and sexual behavior, and are therefore potentially preventable by changes in personal health practices."

Early Warning Signs

(cancer related and otherwise)
If you notice any of these signs, see your doctor promptly.

- A change in urination (more frequent, weaker, painful)
- Blood in urine
- Swollen lymph nodes in the groin area, mild groin pain or unexplained groin bump or swelling that continues for more than one week
- Persistent fever not associated with cold or flu, sweats
- Sudden weight loss
- Chronic fatigue
- Low back pain not associated with injury or trauma
- Swelling of ankles or legs, numbness or weakness of legs
- Pain or itching in the anal area
- Change in bowel habits or in stools, blood in stools
- Unusual or persistent sore, lump, blemish, or marking on the skin
- Change in appearance of a mole
- Nausea or vomiting, pain and tenderness in abdomen

High Blood Pressure

Normal: below 130/85
High-normal: 130-139/85-89
High: over 140/90

High blood pressure is associated with stroke, heart attack, and kidney disease. Some ways to prevent problems with high blood pressure are to lose weight; exercise regularly; reduce the amount of saturated fat and salt in your diet; and get enough potassium (orange juice, potatoes, bananas), calcium (dairy foods, tofu, broccoli, greens, sardines), and magnesium (leafy greens, whole grains); lose weight; limit your alcohol consumption to 2 or fewer drinks per day, and quit smoking.

Cholesterol

Source: The Healthwise Handbook

HDL — "Good Cholesterol"
LDL — "Bad Cholesterol"

	Optimal *All of the following:*	Borderline high-risk *One or more of the following:*	High-risk *One or more of the following:*
Total cholesterol	below 200	200-39	240 or higher
HDL cholesterol	above 35		below 35
LDL cholesterol	below 130	130-59	
Total to HDL ratio	below 3.5	3.5-4.5	4.5 or higher
LDL to HDL ratio	lower than 3		3 or higher

NOTE: *Determining accurate levels of desirable cholesterol depends upon age, gender, and other cardiac risk factors. Every person should consult a physician for his own optimal levels.*

Blood Test Statistics

The following table is a brief aid toward interpreting the results of various blood tests. However, all lab results should be discussed with your doctor or clinician.

	Recommended Levels	Comments
Blood Sugar	GLU (fasting glucose level)-should be 60-126 mg/dl	Higher levels could indicate diabetes
Kidneys	BUN (blood urea nitrogen)-should be 8-23 mg/dl CREAT (creatinine)-should be less than 1.5 mg/dl	Elevated amounts of either BUN or CREAT can signal kidney disease
Liver	BIL (bilirubin count)-should not exceed 1.2 mg/dl ALT (alanine amino transferase)-should not exceed 40 units per liter FER (serum ferritin count)-should be less than 300 mg/ml	Strong variations of BIL or ALT could indicate liver disease, such as cirrhosis A higher FER count could point to hemochromatosis (a disease involving poor iron metabolism)
Prostate	PSA (prostate specific antigen count)-should be less than 4 mcg/l *(Normal levels of PSA are dependent upon age, race, and risk factors)*	A higher level, or a PSA increase of more than 1 mcg/l within a year, should be checked out by a doctor (this is not a standard test)
Blood Cells	WBC (white blood cell count)-should be less than 12,000 per mm^3 RBC (red blood cell count)-should be higher than 4.6 million per mm^3	A higher WBC count might signal infection A lower RBC count could mean a bleeding ulcer or tumor, or iron deficiency
Joints	UA (uric acid)-normal range is 2.4-6 mg/dl	Any more UA (more than 10 mg/dl) may bring on gout, a type of arthritis

Weight

Recent studies by the U.S. National Center for Health show that one third of all adult Americans are overweight; 25% more than 15 years ago. No matter how much media attention is given to fat-free foods, fitness programs, or new exercise machines, Americans continue to eat too many of the wrong foods and to exercise too little. Excess weight can be a factor in many health problems such as heart disease, some cancers, diabetes, high blood pressure, high cholesterol, arthritis, gallstones, and back problems.

It is difficult to determine each individual's ideal weight without considering other factors like body composition (a muscular person may appear to be heavy on the charts), frame size, where the body stores excess fat (fat on the upper body seems to be a greater contributing factor to diabetes, heart disease and high blood pressure), medical and family history, and age (10-15 pounds extra on a person over 70 can be a good thing).

A height and weight table (like the following) can, however be a good starting point.

HEIGHT (Feet, Inches)	WEIGHT		
	Small Frame	Medium Frame	Large Frame
5'2"	128-134 lbs.	131-141 lbs.	138-150 lbs.
5'3"	130-136	133-143	140-153
5'4"	132-138	135-145	142-156
5'5"	134-140	137-148	144-160
5'6"	136-142	139-151	146-164
5'7"	138-145	142-154	149-168
5'8"	140-148	145-157	152-172
5'9"	142-151	148-160	155-176
5'10"	144-154	151-163	158-180
5'11"	146-157	154-166	161-184
6'0"	149-160	157-170	164-188
6'1"	152-164	160-174	168-192
6'2"	155-168	164-178	172-197
6'3"	158-172	167-182	176-202
6'4"	162-176	171-187	181-207

Based on data from the Metropolitan Life Insurance Company, 1983

Body Mass Index

Another way to determine a healthy weight is by calculating your percentage of body fat, measured by the Body Mass Index (BMI). Recommended BMI's are generally in the range of 20-26 (screened area, below).

HEIGHT	WEIGHT									
	130 lbs.	140 lbs.	150 lbs.	160 lbs.	170 lbs.	180 lbs.	190 lbs.	200 lbs.	210 lbs.	220 lbs.
5'4"	22	24	25	27	29	30	32	34		
5'5"	21	23	24	26	28	29	31	33		
5'6"	20	22	24	25	27	29	30	32	33	35
5'7"	20	21	23	25	26	28	29	31	32	34
5'8"	19	21	22	24	25	27	28	30	31	33
5'9"	19	20	22	23	25	26	28	29	31	32
5'10"	18	20	21	22	24	25	27	28	30	30
5'11"	18	19	20	22	23	25	26	27	29	30
6'0"		18	20	21	23	24	25	27	28	29
6'1"		18	19	21	22	23	25	26	27	29
6'2"		17	19	20	21	23	24	25	26	28
6'3"		17	18	19	21	22	23	24	25	27

Calories Burned During Physical Activity

Activity	Calories Burned per hour*
Basketball (full court)	669
Bicycling (6mph)	240
Bicycling (12mph)	410
Gardening	345
Golf (carrying clubs)	340
Jogging (5mph)	740
Running (10mph)	1280
Swimming (50 yds./min)	500
Walking (2 mph)	240
Weight Training	270

*The more you weigh, the more calories you burn. These figures are for a person weighing approximately 150 pounds.

Target Heart Rate

The normal adult resting pulse is 50-100 beats per minute. Your maximum heart rate is figured by subtracting your age from 220. The most aerobic benefit from exercise comes when your heart rate during exercise is 60-80 percent of your maximum heart rate. For example, if you are 40 years old, your maximum heart rate is 180. Therefore, your target exercise heart rate should be 108-144 beats per minute.

Birth Control

TYPE	METHOD	PREGNANCIES (per 100 women per year unless otherwise noted)*	COMMENTS
Surgical	Vasectomy (men)	1/400	Can be reversed only through surgery
	Tubal Ligation (women)	1/200	
Hormonal Methods	Oral (the Pill)	3	Increased risk of circu-latory disorders and high blood pressure; may cause irregular menstrual bleeding
	Norplant (implant)	less than 1	
	Depo-Provera (injection)	less than 1	
IUD (Intra uterine device)		less than 1	May cause bleeding and cramping; may be expelled; increased risk of pelvic infection
Barrier Methods	Condom alone	12	Must be used properly for maximum effectiveness
	Condom with spermicide	5	Most reliable protection against STDs
	Sponge	18-28	Does not protect against STDs
	Diaphragm (with spermicide)	18	Does not protect against STDs
	Cervical cap	18	Does not protect against STDs
Spermicides	Jelly, cream, foam, suppositories (without condom)	21	Use with condom for best protection from pregnancy and STDs
	Used with condom	5	
Periodic Abstinence	Natural methods: tracking body temperature or mucous; rhythm/calendar method	40	
Withdrawal		18	
None		85	

*These rates are lower when the methods are followed perfectly

Sexually Transmitted Diseases

An STD, or sexually transmitted disease, is any disease or infection that is contracted through sexual intercourse or genital contact.

Some of the more serious STDs and venereal diseases (VD) are gonorrhea, syphilis, chlamydia, genital herpes, genital warts, and hepatitis B. AIDS (acquired immuno deficiency syndrome) is the last phase of the disease caused by HIV (human immunodeficiency virus). This virus destroys the human immune system so that the body is unable to fight off even minor diseases or infections.

See your doctor immediately if you notice any of the following symptoms, or if you have reason to believe that you have been exposed to an STD:

- Pain during urination
- Discharge from the penis
- The appearance of painful sores or blisters, or a chancre, on the genitals, or around the mouth or rectum
- Bumps or flat white patches on the penis or scrotum or around the anus
- Vomiting or abdominal pain

- Decrease of appetite or rapid and unexplained weight loss
- Yellow tint to the eyes and skin
- Swollen lymph nodes in the groin area, arm pits, or neck
- Skin rash or patchy hair loss
- Persistent flu-like symptoms
- Fever or night sweats
- Severe chronic fatigue
- Persistent diarrhea

There are many illnesses other than STDs or AIDS that can cause the above symptoms. However, if left untreated, STDs can be very serious; always see your doctor if you have any of these symptoms, especially if your lifestyle or sexual activities put you at risk for infection.

Prevention of STDs

Celibacy or monogamy between uninfected partners is the only way to avoid risk of contracting an STD or HIV. However, following are some ways to reduce the risk of infection and the spread of STDs:

- Avoid all sexual contact during the time that either you or your partner is being treated for an STD of any kind.
- Learn about every partner's lifestyle and sexual history before beginning any sexual relationship to determine if his

or her behavior puts either of you at risk. Use a condom with every partner until you have both been tested, are sure he or she is uninfected, and agree to be monogamous for the duration of your relationship. Remember that it takes up to six months after infection before HIV can be detected in the blood, but that a person may transmit the disease even in the absence of symptoms. Avoid sexual contact with anyone whose behavior or sexual history may not be risk free.

- If you or your partner has herpes, even in the absence of visible symptoms, always use a condom.
- During the presence of any herpes-related sore or blister, avoid sexual contact completely.
- Use latex, not "natural" or lamb-skin condoms from the beginning to the end of sexual contact. Use a spermicide containing nonoxynol-9 in addition to condoms. If the condom does not already have spermicide, apply the spermicide directly into the vagina, not into the condom. Spermicides, the sponge, or the diaphragm do not adequately protect against STDs when used without a condom.

Index

Acknowledgments

The content and creation of this book was shaped with much help from several talented women. I want to thank Meredith Wolf Schizer, Marsha Burns, and Gretchen Scoble for their enthusiasm and excellent work. Susan Costello, Robert Abrams, Patricia Fabricant, and Myrna Smoot also deserve special thanks for keeping the idea rolling. Finally, many individuals have been helpful in offering their suggestions and opinions on simple ways to make men a little more comfortable, attractive, and secure. Thanks to you all.